Surgical Problems in Clinical Practice

Surgical Problems in Clinical Practice

Edited by

John Fry OBE, MD, FRCS, FRCGP
Senior General Practitioner, Beckenham, Kent

Hedley E. Berry MB, BS, FRCS
Consultant Surgeon, King's College Hospital, London and Farnborough Hospital, Kent

Edward Arnold

© Edward Arnold (Publishers) Ltd 1987

First published in Great Britain 1987 by
Edward Arnold (Publishers) Ltd, 41 Bedford Square, London WC1B 3DQ

Edward Arnold (Australia) Pty Ltd, 80 Waverley Road, Caulfield East, Victoria 3145, Australia

Edward Arnold, 3 East Read Street, Baltimore, Maryland 21202, U.S.A.

British Library Cataloguing in Publication Data

Surgical problems in clinical practice.
  1. Diagnosis, Surgical
  I. Fry, John, *1922-*   II. Berry, Hedley E.
  617'.075   RD35

ISBN 0–7131–4504–8

All rights reserved. No part of this publication may be reproduced, stored in a retrieval system, or transmitted in any form or by any means, electronic, photocopying, recording, or otherwise, without the prior permission of Edward Arnold (Publishers) Ltd.

Whilst the advice and information in this book is believed to be true and accurate at the date of going to press, neither the authors nor the publisher can accept any legal responsibility or liability for any errors or omissions that may be made.

Text set in Linotype CRTronic 10/11pt Times
by Anneset, Weston-super-Mare, Avon
Printed in Great Britain by
Butler & Tanner Ltd, London and Frome

Contributors

Hedley E. Berry, MB, BS, FRCS
Department of Surgery
King's College Hospital
Denmark Hill
London
SE5 9RS

John Bradbeer, MA, MB, FRCS
3 Elton Road
Purley
Croydon
Surrey
CR2 3NP

Douglas R. Donaldson, BSc, MD, FRCS, FRCS(Ed)
Department of Surgery
University Hospital of Wales
Heath Park
Cardiff
CF4 4XY

John Fry, OBE, MD, FRCS, FRCGP
138 Croydon Road,
Beckenham
Kent
BR3 4DG

Keith G. Harding, MB, ChB
103 Newport Road
Cardiff
CF2 1AF

Simon Janvrin MS, FRCS
Murrayfield
Gordon Road
Horsham
West Sussex
RH12 2EF

Harold Ludman, MA, FRCS
149 Harley Street
London
W1N 2DE

Brian R. McAvoy, MB, ChB(Hons), BSc(Hons), MRCP, MRCGP
Department of Community Health
Leicester Royal Infirmary
Leicester
LE2 7LZ

Timothy Morley, MA, MB, FRCS
Department of Surgery
King's College Hospital
London
SE5 9RS

Mark M. Orr, BSc, FRCS
Horton General Hospital
Oxford Road
Banbury
Oxon
OX16 9AL

Brian I. Rees, FRCS
St David's
The Avenue
Llandaff
Cardiff

Gillian Strube, MB, BS, DCH
33 Goffs Park Road
Crawley
Sussex
RH11 8AX

M. Keith Thompson, FRCGP
Woodside Health Centre
Enmore Road
London
SE25

Preface

This is an unique book written by the unusual combinations of surgeons and general practitioners combining to present their conjoint views on selected conditions common both in a general practice and in the experience of a district general hospital.

Good surgery now is very much more than demonstrable technical skills carried out by highly trained surgeons. It is a delicate combination of art, science and craft. It is a specialist discipline where practitioners have to work closely with colleagues in other specialties. Of these, general practice is most important, for it is the general practitioner working in the front line of medical care who has the tasks and responsibilities to make the earliest decisions on diagnosis, assessment and management.

The **general practitioner** has to take fundamental decisions on:

what is the likely diagnosis?
what else may it be?
what may happen to the patient (i.e. what is the likely natural history of the disease)?
what to do?
now, instantly
next, in the next few hours
subsequently, over days, weeks and months, if necessary.

The **surgeon** is involved with the middle of a clinical sandwich – concerned with the more definitive assessment, diagnosis and treatment, before passing the patient back to the general practitioner.

For optimal care both *general practitioner and surgeon* must understand each others problems, skills and contributions. The general practitioner must know about what is necessary and what is possible in modern surgery. The surgeon must be concerned with teaching, informing and updating his general practitioner colleagues on what can and what cannot be expected from modern surgery.

Our aims have been to present to general practitioners the experienced views of surgeons and to give surgeons an insight into some of the problems faced by general practitioners.

Although we hope that all general practitioners and surgeons will find much to make them reflect, and much to apply, our chief targets are the coming generations of general practitioner trainees, surgical housemen and registrars, and more senior medical students about to embark on their final examinations.

1986

H.E.B.
J.F.

Contents

Preface		vi
1	**Basics**	1
	Hedley E. Berry and John Fry	
2	**Surgical Problems in Children**	4
	Brian I. Rees, Douglas R. Donaldson and Keith G. Harding	
3	**Ear, Nose and Throat Conditions**	15
	Harold Ludman and John Fry	
4	**Lumps in the Neck**	38
	Hedley E. Berry and John Fry	
5	**Thyroid Disorders**	47
	Hedley E. Berry and John Fry	
6	**Lumps in the Breast**	57
	John Bradbeer and M. Keith Thompson	
7	**The Abdomen:** Acute and Chronic Disorders	68
	Simon Janvrin and Gillian Strube	
8	**Herniae and Scrotal Swellings**	78
	Mark M. Orr and Brian R. McAvoy	
9	**Jaundice**	93
	John Bradbeer and M. Keith Thompson	
10	**Low Back Pain**	102
	Timothy Morley and John Fry	
11	**Varicose Veins and their Effects**	111
	Mark M. Orr and Brian R. McAvoy	
12	**The Ischaemic Leg**	123
	Mark M. Orr and Brian R. McAvoy	
Index		137

1 Basics

Hedley E. Berry and John Fry

What is surgery?

Surgery is more than a technical procedure – the real skills lie in early diagnosis, the selection of the patients and the selection of the operation.

Complete care demands co-operation between surgeon and general practitioner at all stages.

Making the clinical diagnosis
Time and expense are saved if the general practitioner carries out appropriate investigations before referral to the surgeon.

Investigation of the patient
Use and misuse of investigations. Sophisticated techniques – CT scanning, isotope scanning are available. It is seldom necessary for a laparotomy to be performed to establish diagnosis. Parathyroid tumours can now be localized with increasing accuracy.

Managing the condition, the patient and the family
The general practitioner is responsible for the initial important decision of deciding optimal treatment – should the patient be referred for surgical opinion or managed conservatively at home?

Discuss and explain with the patient and family. The general practitioner must know the basic steps involved in surgical treatment so that the patient can be informed and reassured. Advice on postoperative recovery and convalescence is based on his knowledge.

When will the patient be fit for work?

Knowledge of surgical procedures is essential for *carrying out after-care*. Hospital stays are shorter and shorter and Day Surgery is increasing. The policy is now to transfer care to the home from the hospital; this leads to increasing involvement of the general practitioner in postoperative care, and the need to recognize postoperative complications such as wound infections if and when they occur; pelvic abscesses complicating appendicitis now often present at home because of this policy of early discharge.

Long-term follow-up surveillance
Ideally this is best done by the general practitioner. After malignant disease, a six-monthly follow-up at the hospital outpatient department is of little value.

Example

Graves disease

Post-thyroidectomy check, because 1 per cent per year become hypothyroid.

Antigen estimations may enable recurrence of malignant disease to be predicted.

Basic needs

The practice of clinical skills in surgery, as in any field of health care, requires much more than the laying-on of hands and the ordering of battery investigations. The basic needs require a broad understanding of the following:

The *nature (pathology)* of the condition

Example

Parotid swellings

70 per cent benign
30 per cent malignant.

The *epidemiology*
The extent and likely frequency – how many cases can be expected in a year?

2 Basics

> *Example*
>
> Annual prevalence in a general practice of 2500 persons
>
> cancers of large bowel 2–3
> cancers of breast 2–3

Distribution – geographical, social, sex, age, etc.

> *Example*
>
> **Duodenal ulcer**
>
> M > F
> peak incidence 20–50 years
> social class 1 > 5.

Risk factors – what makes prognosis worse?

> *Example*
>
> **Appendicitis**
>
> young and old fare worse.

Possibilities for prevention.

> *Example*
>
> mammography may reduce mortality from breast cancer by 30 per cent (by early diagnosis).

The natural history

What is likely to happen to the patient over the next few weeks, months, years. The patient and family will want to know.

> *Example*
>
> **Cancer 5 year survival (%)**
>
> | | |
> |---|---|
> | testis | 67 |
> | breast | 57 |
> | large bowel | 33 |
> | stomach | 7 |

Diagnostic procedures
Importance of the *history*

> *Example*
>
> The distinction of irritable bowel syndrome from a more serious pathology (cancer) rests on the assessment history by GP, and on selection of cases for further investigation.

Clinical examination (supportive evidence)

> *Example*
>
> more errors arise from failure to examine the patient than from any other factor.
>
> abdominal conditions cannot be diagnosed by telephone.
>
> management of abdominal pain often depends on physical signs.
>
> repeated examination often necessary, e.g. breast 'lump' after menstrual period and abdominal pain after a few hours.

Questions and answers

What may it be?
How does it present and why?
Who gets it when?
What may happen?
What to do and who does what?
What outcomes?

In all forms of care by general practitioners and surgeons a process of 'self-checking' should be carried out to review failures as well as successes.

Collaboration

Good care of surgical patients depends on good liaison, understanding and collaboration between general practitioners and surgeons. Each must respect the other and be familiar with each other's problems and difficulties. The general practitioner must know the policies of referral and management in local surgical units and in particular the detailed steps for cases such as 'breast lumps,' 'piles,' (rectal bleeding) and 'the acute abdomen'; how to arrange urgent referrals; how to live with long waiting lists, rationing and priorities.

It is the general practitioner who has to decide on degrees of urgency and priority.

The surgeon must appreciate the nature of general practice and the practitioner's difficulties in assessing the case at the earliest stages and having to make decisions on possible diagnosis, on whether to treat the patient at home or to admit, and on how long is it justifiable to wait for an outpatient consultation appointment.

The place of the domiciliary consultation should be recognized. This is particularly useful in the difficult subacute abdomen, in the elderly and disabled, and for support of families in caring for the dying at home.

2 Surgical Problems in Children

Brian I. Rees, Douglas R. Donaldson, Keith G. Harding

Children requiring admission to hospital should be admitted to a paediatric ward; as three-quarters of those children needing an operation will have it performed by a general surgeon, close co-operation with the paediatrician is essential. The majority of children admitted for surgical reasons will need to stay in hospital for one or two nights or less.

Older children can be regarded physiologically as young adults whereas neonates and young children cannot. A 3.5 kg neonate has a plasma volume of only 140 ml and the loss of gastric contents and/or diarrhoea can quickly result in dehydration. Babies are particularly sensitive to heat loss because of their large surface area relative to size, and during transportation of a neonate to hospital precautions must be taken to minimize heat loss, for example by the use of incubators.

Whether a child is seen at home or in the general practitioner's surgery, a working diagnosis has to be made. Having established a diagnosis the practitioner now decides if the child can be managed at home or should be referred to a hospital. If referral to a hospital is necessary, should this be as an emergency or can the child be seen in the outpatient department? We will discuss some of the more common surgical problems encountered in practice and hope to give some guidelines in their management.

Common surgical conditions in children

Requiring emergency admission

Head injury
Acute abdominal pain
Vomiting in the newborn
Abscesses
Burns
Incarcerated hernia

Requiring elective admission

Phimosis – see section on GU tract
Hernias
Genitourinary tract conditions
Undescended testis – see section on GU tract
Neck/facial swellings
Birthmarks
   hare-lip/cleft palate

Conditions requiring emergency admission
Head injury

This is a major cause of serious disability and death in childhood. Admissions for head injury form 6.7 per cent of total hospital admissions for 0–14-year-olds.

Presentation
The majority present directly to casualty, but some will inevitably be seen initially by the general practitioner.

Causes
   Road-traffic accidents
   Falls from heights
   Playground equipment accidents, e.g. swings.

Symptoms
   Variable but include:
      unconsciousness
      drowsiness

nausea/vomiting
blurred vision
irritability
fits
headaches.

There is a good correlation between the severity of head injury and the extent of retrograde amnesia.

Management

If there is any doubt in the clinician's mind, or if symptoms suggest significant injury, hospital admission for a period of observation is mandatory. Open head injuries, overt skull fractures, and CSF rhinorrhoea or otorrhoea require immediate hospital admission. The comatose child with a severe head injury must have his airway maintained and be moved as little as possible, in view of the risk of other injuries including fractures of the spine.

Sequelae of head injury
Herniation of brain tissue through fracture sites
Leakage of CSF
Extradural haematoma
Subdural haematoma
Intracerebral haematoma
Infections
Epilepsy (10 per cent of children develop epilepsy following head injury)
Irritability and impairment of concentration

Prognosis of head injuries
Complete recovery	85%
Death	10%
Recovery with a significant neurological deficit	5%

Head Injury

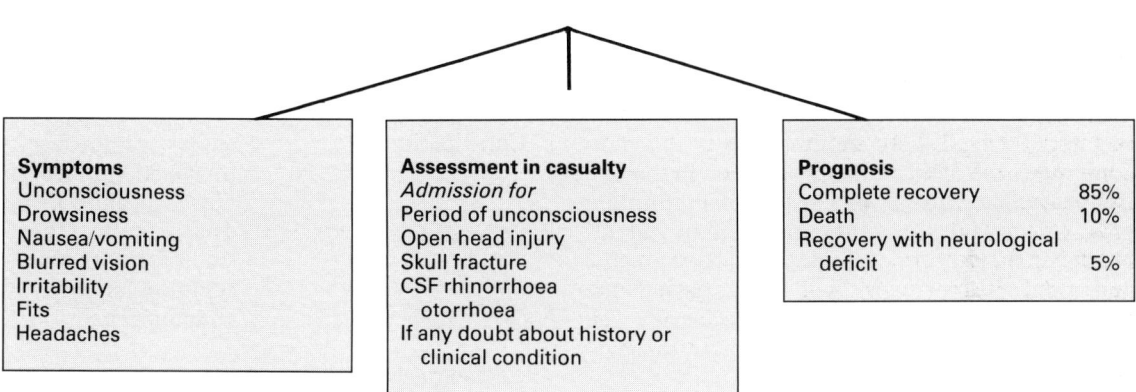

Symptoms
Unconsciousness
Drowsiness
Nausea/vomiting
Blurred vision
Irritability
Fits
Headaches

Assessment in casualty
Admission for
Period of unconsciousness
Open head injury
Skull fracture
CSF rhinorrhoea
 otorrhoea
If any doubt about history or clinical condition

Prognosis
Complete recovery 85%
Death 10%
Recovery with neurological
 deficit 5%

Acute abdominal pain

Acute abdominal pain is a very common condition presenting to the family doctor, and whilst in the majority of patients the pain will settle spontaneously, a significant number will either be admitted to hospital immediately or after a period of observation.

Appendicitis

This is the cause of 18/1000 patients consulting per year. Children may present with typical features of appendicitis, but often the history and physical findings are not typical; nevertheless a high index of suspicion should lead the doctor to suspect the diagnosis in children who present with abdominal pain.

Differential diagnosis

Gastrointestinal	appendicitis
	Meckel's diverticulum
	gastroenteritis
	constipation
	Henoch–Schönlein
	purpura
Liver and gall bladder	hepatitis
	gall stones

Pancreas	pancreatitis cystic fibrosis
Renal	urinary tract infection renal calculi
Spleen	splenic infarction
Lymph	mesenteric adenitis

Treatment

In children clinical suspicion is the usual major factor in deciding to operate, and although biochemical and radiological tests may assist they are not invariably helpful and appendicectomy is usually performed in the acute stage of the illness; only very rarely is an appendix abscess seen today; this is then treated conservatively and the patient undergoes elective appendicectomy at a later date.

Intussusception

This occurs in 2/1000 live births; it is most common in children aged 4–12 months and is the most common cause of intestinal obstruction in the first two years. There usually is a history of intermittent colic arising unexpectedly in a healthy infant. However, 10 per cent of children will have no pain and only 50 per cent will have passed the 'redcurrant' bloody stool. The child is usually well between spasms when the diagnostic sausage-shaped mass is felt.

There is occasionally a local cause for the problem, e.g. a Meckel's diverticulum, or polyp which is usually found in the ileocolic region.

In a number of cases it is possible to reduce the intussusception hydrostatically by the use of a barium enema, but there remains a risk of recurrence. Attempts at hydrostatic reduction should not be made when symptoms have been present for more than 48 hours or where there is evidence of peritonism.

Chronic and recurrent abdominal pains

This is seen in 10 per cent of schoolchildren, and no organic cause is found in 90 per cent of cases. Usually reassurance is all that is necessary, but it is important to identify those suffering with organic causes, which are:

Urinary tract infection	investigate with urine cultures and ultrasound, followed by more specialist radiology where indicated.
Peptic ulcer	rare, but does occur in children; barium meal.
Inflammatory bowel disease	change of bowel habit, will need barium meal and follow-through, barium enema and sigmoidoscopy.
Constipation	exclude organic causes for constipation, e.g. Hirschsprung's disease; culture the stools for worms, a common cause of abdominal pain.

Each attack of abdominal pain may result in hospital admission and increase both the child's and the parents' anxieties. When there is no apparent cause for the abdominal pain, calm reassurance should be applied.

Children who do not have an organic cause for their abdominal pain often progress into adulthood still suffering from recurrent attacks.

Note that:
'Little belly achers become big belly achers.'

Vomiting in the newborn

Bile-stained vomiting in a neonate should be regarded as due to intestinal obstruction until proven otherwise. The majority of such cases are due to a congenital bowel obstruction (atresia or stenosis of the bowel, malrotation, congenital bands), which is usually below the level of the ampulla of Vater – hence the bile-stained vomit. A small percentage of cases will be due to Hirschsprung's disease, and in only 20–25 per cent will no cause be found. All neonates with bile vomiting must be admitted to hospital.

In first few months

Vomiting in the first few months is usually due to feeding difficulties. The child is sick after every feed (often with wind) but looks well. The mother needs constant reassurance in such circumstances, with help from the Health Visitor.

Congenital hypertrophic pyloric stenosis
This occurs in the first few months of life, commonly between 4 and 6 weeks. The vomiting is regular and projectile and can be blood stained due to an associated gastritis. There is often a family history; it occurs in a male:female ratio of 4:1, and is more common in firstborn infants.

The child is restless, persistently hungry, looks unwell, may have visible peristalsis, and a pyloric tumour may be felt whilst the child feeds. Treatment of this condition is by division of the hypertrophied muscle fibres of the pylorus (pyloromyotomy), and usually leads to a rapid improvement. Any child with persistent vomiting needs hospital admission.

In older children

This may be a feature of any illness, but when due to intestinal obstruction is usually associated with abdominal pain and constipation. The differential diagnosis includes infections (otitis media and tonsillitis) allergies, poisoning, intracranial space-occupying lesions, and emotional upset.

Abscesses

These occur in 3.5/1000 patients of 0–15 years of age.

They usually occur as a result of secondary infection of the lymphoid tissue (therefore the cervical and axillary nodes are common sites) and are often associated with upper respiratory tract infections which have cleared or been treated with antibiotics before the nodes became enlarged.

Other sites of infection are the groin, breast, perianal area, or umbilicus.

Rare causes of abscess formation are tuberculous lymphadenitis or underlying osteomyelitis.

Treatment
If the diagnosis is in doubt, needle aspiration by a skilled person may be necessary to ensure that the correct diagnosis is made. If the lesion is not progressing towards resolution after a period of observation or with appropriate antibiotics, surgical drainage or excision should be undertaken.

It should be added that lymphadenopathy in children can persist for a very long time in a healthy child, and is usually of no significance.

Burns

Burns result in 0.7 per cent of all hospital admissions for children under 14 years of age, with an average hospital stay of 12–14 days.

Causes
Scalds. From hot liquids; commonly seen in children under three years of age.
Flame burns. Clothing is ignited, often when the child stands too close to a source of heat.
Hot-metal burns. Usually on the hands, often from grasping something hot, e.g. an electric fire.
Friction burns. From ropes or playground equipment, or following accidents.

Factors to consider
Area of burns. If more than 10 per cent of the body surface is burnt, the child should be in hospital.
Depth of burns. The simplest classification is 'partial' or 'full thickness', but there is no universal classification.

Remember. The fluid loss is greatest in the first 24 hours, and a deep burn area is anaesthetic.

Dressings
Occlusion. If this method is used, dressing should not macerate or damage tissues, and should be

padded sufficiently to prevent exudate soaking through to the surface.

Exposure. Normally used for superficial burns. Exudate dries in 48–72 hours, then crusts and lifts off in 14–21 days.

Healing. Superficial burns heal within 10–21 days. *Deep burns* require grafting, and healing times are variable, depending on the number of grafts needed to cover the defect.

Complications

Infections. Burns are particularly prone to infection by:
Staphylococcus aureus
Streptococcus pyogenes
Pseudomonas aeruginosa.

Burns

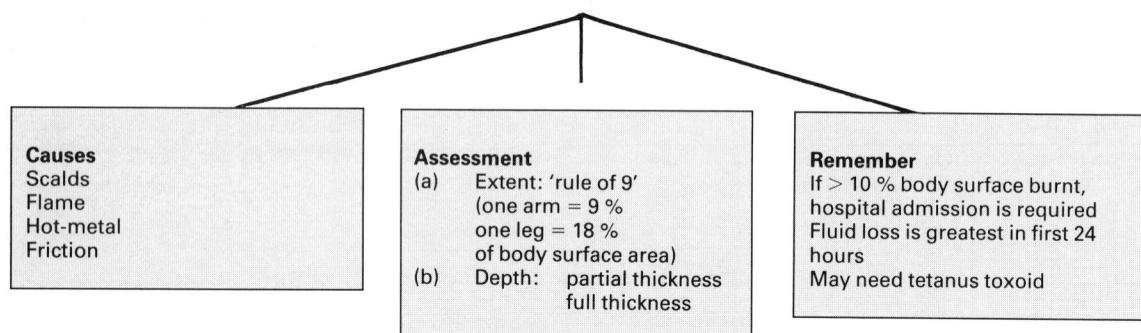

Reduce infection by good nursing and dressing care. Use of silver sulphadiazine (Flamazine) in dressings.

Contractures
The early advice of a plastic surgeon is required to prevent the occurrence of contractures.

Hypertrophic scars
These too should be seen and assessed by a plastic surgeon.

Conditions requiring elective admission
Hernia (See also page 80)

Inguinal hernias. These are common in infancy and due to a patent processus vaginalis; they are more common in boys but can be seen in girls. They can be unilateral or bilateral. When the groin swellings are bilateral in girls the possibility that they are testicles should be considered, and a chromosome count may be necessary.

The inguinal hernia can present as an intermittent groin swelling, seen when the child plays or strains, or as a lump that appears and does not go down. The possibility of an incarcerated hernia should be considered. This requires immediate referral to hospital as an *emergency*. With an intermittent groin swelling an urgent outpatient appointment should be sought.

When a child has an *incarcerated hernia* and there is no evidence of strangulation (painful swelling, signs of intestinal obstruction) then the child should be given a sedative and (a) placed in gallows, or (b) the foot end of the bed should be elevated to allow spontaneous reduction. This can be tried over a few hours. If the swelling does not reduce, proceed to operation. Taxis (reduction by applying pressure to the swelling) should only be performed by an experienced paediatrician or surgeon. If the hernia reduces, it is the practice of most surgeons to place the patient on the next convenient surgical list for herniotomy.

Regardless of the patient's age, all inguinal hernias in children require operation – herniotomy (ligation of the sac), for they all potentially risk incarceration and strangulation. With advances in anaesthesia, *it is not necessary to wait for the child to reach a certain age.*

Umbilical hernia. This is common, particularly in black children; there are two different types.

The true umbilical hernia is through the central cicatrix and is common. It is a bulge which pushes the overlying umbilical skin straight out. The hernia is easily reduced, and even quite large defects can undergo spontaneous resolution. The hernia is painless and strangulation virtually unknown; all that is necessary is reassurance to the mother.

However, the *supra-umbilical* hernia is a defect in the linea alba through which omentum or small bowel herniate. The swelling points downwards. It will not heal spontaneously and should be closed at about four years of age.

Epigastric hernia. This is usually noted by parents as a swelling in the midline which is painless. It is the result of a small defect in the linea alba, and the swelling is usually a small amount of preperitoneal fat. The hernia will not disappear and should be referred as a non-urgent case for repair.

Inguinal hernia/hydrocele

Pathophysiology
Patent processus vaginalis
Hernia nearly always indirect
Incidence ♂ : ♀ = 10:1
50 per cent may be bilateral

Presentation
Hernia
  'Lump in groin or scrotum'
  often intermittent
  cannot get above it
  risk of strangulation
Hydrocele
  scrotal swelling
  can usually get above it
Both may
  transilluminate

Course and prognosis
Hernia
  risk of strangulation
  never regresses
  ∴ refer for operation
Hydrocele
  < 1 year, usually regresses
  > 1 year, tense, refer for operation

Genitourinary tract conditions

Enuresis

This can be divided into primary and secondary.

Primary
(The child has never been dry)
  Causes in the female: ectopic opening of urethra in vagina
              ectopic ureter
  in the male: ectopic ureter
          urethral obstruction
          (urethral valves)
          urethral diverticulum
  in either: (neurogenic)
         meningocele
         agenesis of sacrum
         delay in maturation of CNS.

Secondary
(The child has dry periods and relapses)
This is usually due to psychological reasons but a urinary tract infection must be excluded.

Persistent enuresis requires investigation and referral to either a paediatrician or a paediatric surgeon/urologist. Most cases are secondary and will respond to counselling, 'wet alarms' and bladder training. It is as well to remember that up to 5 per cent of children will not be dry at ten years of age.

Urinary tract infections

To establish the diagnosis of UTI one must ensure that the specimen is not contaminated. This requires not only the swabbing of the external genitalia, but retraction of the foreskin in boys and the holding apart of the labia in girls.

Symptoms are often non-specific in the younger child, who may present with failure to thrive, vomiting, recurrent fever or recurrent abdominal pain. Haematuria can occasionally occur but is more commonly associated with tuberculosis, angioma or, rarely, with Wilm's tumour. Tuberculosis should be suspected if a sterile pyuria is repeatedly found, with no growth on ordinary culture.

A definite UTI in a child should be investigated with at least an IVP to exclude stasis. Stasis may be caused by:

obstruction to the lower urinary tract
posterior urethral valves
urethral stricture
urethral diverticulum
Marion's disease (bladder-neck obstruction)

obstruction to the upper urinary tract
hydronephrosis
ureterocele
retrocaval ureter

neuropathy
spina bifida
sacral agenesis.

vesicoureteric reflux
This is the most common cause and is usually due to a primary defect at the ureteric orifice. The ureter becomes dilated and eventually the renal pelvis will dilate; the renal parenchyma becomes progressively destroyed. Reflux may be secondary to obstruction in the lower urinary tract. If this is present reimplantation of the ureter may have to be considered.

Penile abnormalities (Figure 2.1)

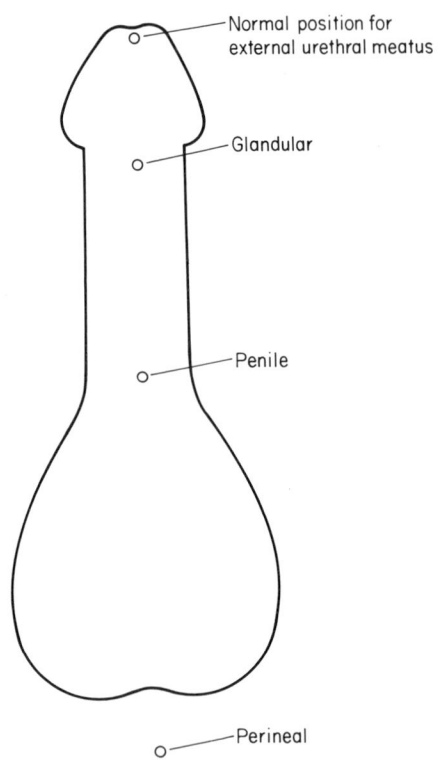

Figure 2.1 Hypospadias.

Hypospadias
occurs in 1:300 male births
most cases are minor
5 per cent have an associated urinary tract abnormality
glandular, penile, and perineal positions are seen.

Glandular
external urinary meatus is in the coronal sulcus
hooded glans
majority need no treatment unless there is spraying of urine or meatal stenosis.

Penile
usually some degree of chordee
surgery necessary in two stages – chordee

corrected at 18 months, 2nd stage at 4 years old involves a strip of skin being buried as a tube.

Perineal
may be confused with intersex state
have severe chordee of penis
phallus may be inadequate for sexual function.

Epispadias
defect lies on the dorsum of the penis
can involve the posterior urethral valve and, therefore, the child may be incontinent
surgery deferred until 3–4 years old so as to assess continence.

Conditions requiring **Circumcision** (Note that 90 per cent of prepuces will retract by two years of age.)

Balanitis Ammoniacal dermatitis affecting the prepuce from the outside is often confused with balanitis; it is not an indication for circumcision. Advise the parents to leave their baby without a napkin and expose the napkin area.
   True balanitis is due to infection of the subprepucial pocket giving a suppurative discharge with swelling of the surrounding tissues. These children often have a non-retractable prepuce.

Phimosis This can result from recurrent attacks of true balanitis, or from fissures due to the forceful stretching and retraction of the foreskin by the parents. This practice is to be condemned.

Paraphimosis Prompt reduction by pulling the tight foreskin distally whilst simultaneously exerting pressure on the glans penis in a proximal direction can obviate hospital admission.

If reduction is not possible, the child requires admission for either a dorsal slit or circumcision.

Religious reasons

Parental pressures 'Both my father and I had it done.'

Undescended testis (Figure 2.2)

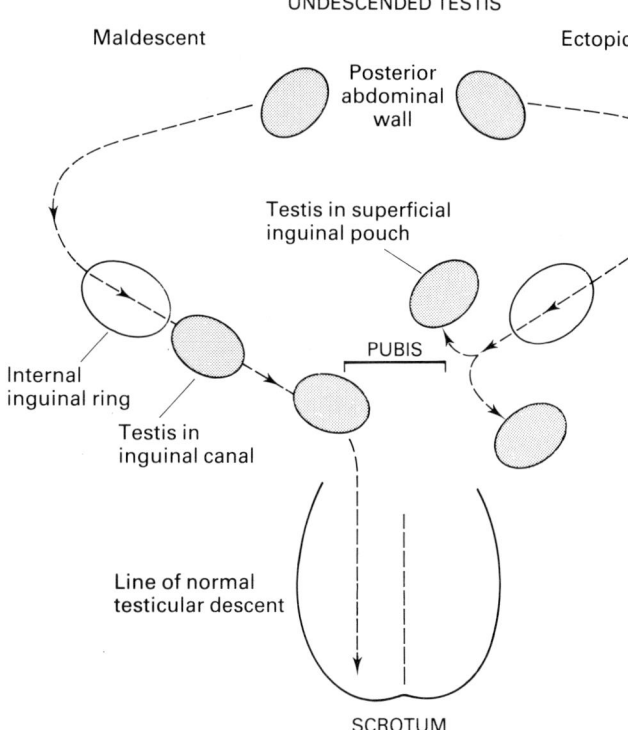

Figure 2.2 Undescended testis.

Maldescent
The testicle lies in the normal line of testicular descent but fails to reach the scrotum.

Ectopic
The testicle is not in the line of normal descent

A common site is the superficial inguinal pouch, anterior to the inguinal canal

Other, rarer, sites include perineal, femoral and prepubic areas.

It is important to differentiate a retractile from an undescended testis. One does this by the squat or chair test. Ask the child to sit on a chair with his feet on the chair and to pull his knees up to his chest. Both these manoeuvres relax the cremasteric reflex, allowing a retractile testis to descend spontaneously, or to be coaxed down with gentle pressure, into the scrotum. If the testis can be thus brought down, surgery is not required as spontaneous normal development and descent will be complete at puberty.

If the testis is truly undescended then orchidopexy is required and is performed in most centres at the age of four or five years, with some centres doing it earlier. This is thought to improve subsequent fertility (virility would usually be unaffected if the testis is left in situ). Repair of the associated inguinal hernia, present in 50 per cent of cases, is also carried out.

An undescended testis is also more likely to undergo malignant transformation (roughly 30 times the risk of a normal scrotal testis).

Swellings of the head and neck (See also Chapter 4)

Only the more common conditions seen in childhood will be dealt with in this section.

External angular dermoid

The lateral end of the eyebrow is a common site for the development of this cystic swelling which is caused by epidermal cells separating at the points of embryological fusion sites. The condition presents as a small swelling which can increase in size slowly. If it becomes infected an abscess can form and recurrent infections may ensue.

Swelling of the parotid

It is unusual to see unilateral swelling of the parotid in children. Bilateral swelling of the parotid area is usually due to mumps. When unilateral swelling occurs and the gland is not tender, the possibility of a parotid haemangioma should be considered. Chronic or recurrent parotitis is not uncommon. The history is of recurrent swellings in one or both cheeks in the parotid area. The gland is tender and there is pain on opening the mouth. It is possible to express drops of pus or turbid fluid from the parotid duct inside the cheek. The organism is usually *Streptococcus viridans* or *Str. pneumoniae*. Treatment of chronic parotitis is with systemic antibiotics and these sometimes have to be continued for several weeks.

Ranula

This is a cystic swelling of the mucous gland in the floor of the mouth. It is treated by surgical deroofing if the symptoms cause discomfort or drooling.

Thyroglossal cyst and sinus

The thyroglossal tract runs from the foramen caecum of the tongue to the region of the hyoid bone and just below it, along the track of the developing thyroid gland. A cystic swelling in the midline of the neck which moves on protrusion of the tongue is usually a thyroglossal cyst. The cyst can become infected, form an abscess, and rupture onto the skin to form a thyroglossal sinus. When making a diagnosis of thyroglossal cyst, consideration should be given as to whether the cyst could be ectopic thyroid tissue, and some authorities advocate a thyroid scan prior to excision. Such a scan will obviate the excision of tissue, which if it is the only functioning thyroid tissue would render the patient myxoedematous. The treatment of a thyroglossal cyst and fistula is excision.

Branchial fistula

The lesion commonly called a branchial fistula is a persistent tract of the second branchial cleft, of which the outer end is covered by the operculum to form the cervical sinus. A small pinpoint orifice in the lower third of the neck at the anterior border of the sternomastoid muscle is easily diagnosed as a branchial fistula. It usually gives no trouble apart from a small discharge of clear mucus; if the fistula becomes infected then an unpleasant discharge of pus can occur. The usual treatment is excision of the complete tract. Occasionally there is only a short tract and this can be associated with a piece of cartilage at its base (accessory auricle). Occasionally only a section of the complete tract persists and this develops into a branchial cyst. The typical branchial cyst presents as a swelling under the angle of the jaw extending in front of and under the sternomastoid muscle. It is usually fluctuant and has been described as feeling like a half-full hot-water bottle. These cysts can become infected and increase in size rapidly. Treatment is by excision.

Cystic hygroma

This is a multilocular malformation of the lymphatics and is most commonly seen in the neck, although it may be seen in the axilla, chest, groins or buttocks. The lymphatic vessels become distended and form a soft swelling which is usually not tender. The mass can vary in size from very small to very large – so large that it can cause compression symptoms. Treatment is by excision, and this has to be done with great care because the lesion is often associated intimately with nerves and vessels.

Lymphadenopathy

Swelling of the lymph nodes in the neck of children is very common and usually secondary to infection. The lymph nodes are tender and will disappear (although not always completely) when the infection has subsided. If a single lymph node becomes enlarged and is non-tender, this should be excised for histology, since as in adults this could be due to Hodgkin's disease or the allied reticuloses. When a swelling in the neck is tender and red it may be an abscess which requires surgical drainage.

Tuberculous cervical lymphadenitis is now rare but still does occur. When excising glands in the neck always consider this diagnosis so that appropriate bacteriology can be obtained.

Birth marks

Capillary haemangioma
A 'strawberry naevus'. This is a raised capillary lesion in the skin.

It usually resolves spontaneously but in certain sites, e.g. on the lip or eyelid, it may need treatment. Constant reassurance to the parent is necessary. Surgical excision is sometimes indicated, and where the lesion is large this may have to be a staged procedure.

Cavernous haemangioma
This may or may not be associated with an overlying birth mark on the skin.

Again, it may resolve spontaneously or respond to injection.

If large, arteriovenous shunting may occur with ensuing cardiac failure.

Capillary naevus
A 'port wine' stain is salmon pink or a dusky hue. If in the distribution of the third cranial nerve, the Sturge-Kalischer-Weber syndrome should be considered; this is a cutaneous lesion associated with an intracranial haemangioma, and the latter can give rise to convulsions and hemiplegia.

Treatment of a capillary naevus is by the use of cosmetic creams rather than plastic procedures unless the lesions are small and easily excised.

Cystic hygroma (lymphangioma)
The cervical region is a common site
A chest x-ray is mandatory to ensure there is no mediastinal extension
Treatment is by surgical excision and suction drainage.

Pigmented naevi
May have hair if mature
Malignant melanoma is extremely rare in childhood
Surgery will be for cosmetic reasons only
May need serial excisions.

Angiomatous or pigmented swellings over the midline of the back should raise the possibility of spina bifida, or, if over the sacrum, of sacrococcygeal teratoma.

Hare lip/cleft palate

There is a range from a notched lip at one extreme to a cleft uvula at the other, with varying degrees of expression up to a complete and bilateral cleft lip and palate.

Cleft lip
The incidence is 1 in 750 live births

   male > female

   left > right

Cleft palate

The incidence is 1 in 2000 live births

    female > male

    cleft palate prevents normal suckling

The child is prone to otitis media and its complications due to the Eustachian tube being wide open and mucus stagnating in the nasopharynx

A major problem is in feeding.

Special teats can be used having a rubber flange above the nipple which closes the gap in the palate.

Treatment

Hare lip is repaired at three months or when child weighs 4.5 kg.

Cleft palate is usually a two-stage procedure. The soft palate is closed when the child is six months old. The hard palate is closed when the child is aged 4–5 years. Some centres close both the soft and hard palate at the same time when the child is aged 12–18 months.

Two-thirds of patients aged 5–13 years with cleft palates will have loss of hearing due to drainage problems of the middle ear, leading to recurrent ear infections. Therefore, all infections should be treated promptly and the eardrum inspected regularly.

Three-quarters of children with cleft palates will speak normally. Their ability to do this depends largely on the surgical success of the soft-palate closure, and on normal hearing. Speech therapy may be required.

At a later date orthodontic and cosmetic surgery may be required.

3 Ear, Nose and Throat Conditions

Harold Ludman and John Fry

Introduction

Diseases of the upper respiratory tract, the ear, nose and throat, are the most widespread group of diseases in the community.

It is the general practitioner, or whoever is the doctor of first contact, who has to make the initial assessment and diagnosis and decide what he/she can manage and what needs to be referred to a specialist.

The approach has to be clinical and practical, and that approach is followed in this chapter. The symptoms and problems selected are those that can cause special difficulties in management.

Ear diseases

Earache and deafness are the most frequent symptoms of ear disease. Giddiness (vertigo; page 22) and facial paralysis (page 25) may be related to disorders in the ears.

Earache; pain in the ear

The most likely cause of earache is inflammation of outer or middle ear and differentiation may be difficult.

Acute otitis externa
This may be diffuse, or localized as a furuncle. A furuncle is very tender and presents in the outer ear canal (Figure 3.1) – there are no hair follicles in the bony meatus. Hearing becomes impaired only if the meatus is blocked by swelling or discharge, and fever occurs only if infection spreads to the skin around the ear as a cellulitis or erysipelas. In those circumstances there may be tender, enlarged nodes palpable in front of or behind the ear, but the tenderness is superficial, unlike that on deep pressure in acute otitis media. The pinna is tender on movement. Any discharge is thick and scanty, unlike the copious mucoid discharge of a middle-ear infection.

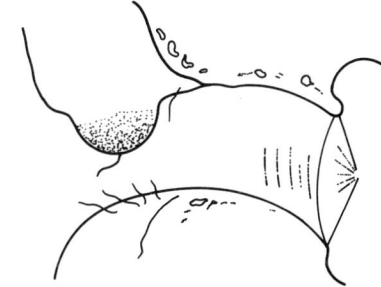

Figure 3.1 A furuncle.

Acute otitis media
Acute otitis media causes deep-seated pain, deafness, and systemic illness with fever. The sequence of symptoms is first a blocked feeling in the ear, pain and fever, followed by discharge

when and if the tympanic membrane perforates, with relief of the pain and fever. In children of course there may not be a clear history of deafness before the onset of pain. The whole middle-ear cleft is affected, so there is always tenderness on deep pressure over the mastoid antrum; this does not imply mastoiditis (Figure 3.2). Diagnosis is made by inspecting the tympanic membrane, but this may be impossible because of wax or meatal wall swelling. Only if the whole drum can be seen to be normal and there is no conductive hearing loss can otitis media be excluded. Lymph nodes in front of or behind the ear are never enlarged in simple otitis media. If there is any doubt about distinguishing acute otitis externa from acute otitis media, it is safer from the practical point of view to treat the condition with systemic antibiotics as acute otitis media. Several attempts at ear-drum inspection may be necessary before a diagnosis can be established firmly.

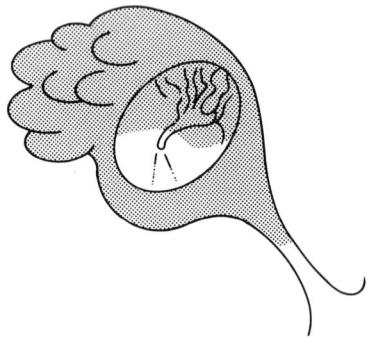

Figure 3.2 Acute otitis media.

Secretory otitis media

Known as 'glue ears', also causes middle-ear inflammatory pain in children who are not suffering from acute otitis media. Their complaint is usually of a short-lasting, niggly pain recurring from time to time, without fever. The appearances of the tympanic membrane may be misleading (Figure 3.3) since injected vessels are often seen with secretory otitis media, and many such children are incorrectly diagnosed as suffering from acute suppurative otitis media.

Glue ears and grommets

Very large numbers of children of school age suffer temporary conductive deafness because of the development of glue ears. This condition should be suspected in any child with an acquired hearing loss, especially if it tends to vary in severity from time to time. It should also be suspected when a child complains of intermittent, frequent, short-lasting pain, and when a tympanic membrane fails to return to normal two or three weeks after an attack of acute suppurative otitis media. All such children will be referred for an ENT opinion. If the effusions have persisted for more than six weeks, the conventional methods of treatment will be by aspiration of the effusion under an anaesthetic, and insertion of a ventilation tube (a grommet; Figure 3.4). This procedure will sometimes be associated with removal of enlarged adenoids, but the role of adenoidectomy in preventing recurrence of effusions is not yet established.

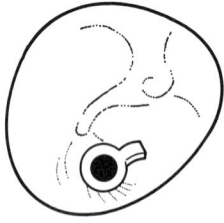

Figure 3.4 A grommet in place.

Conventional ventilation tubes or grommets are extruded from the tympanic membrane and pushed out with wax along the external auditory meatus. The period of time from insertion of a grommet until it becomes blocked and therefore ineffective varies from three months to over a year. If a grommet becomes blocked there is a risk, affecting 30 per cent of children in whom grommets are inserted, that the effusions will recur. If that happens it may be necessary to insert another grommet, and on occasions ventilation tubes of a design which will enable them to remain in place for several years are inserted (Figure 3.5).

The matter of grommets and swimming is

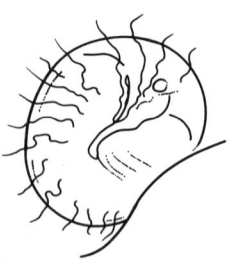

Figure 3.3 Secretory otitis media.

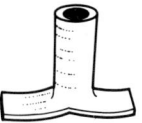

Figure 3.5 A grommet for long-term use.

controversial. It is now known that the risk of water passing through the lumen of a conventional grommet (0.8 mm) is very small. Under raised pressure the risk is greater, so if children do swim they must be persuaded to keep to the surface. Unfortunately the problem of swimming and grommets is not confined merely to that of water passing into the middle ear. There seems no doubt that the chemical irritation of chlorinated water acting on the nasopharyngeal end of the Eustachian tube provokes middle-ear infections, and predisposes to reformation of middle-ear effusions. For these reasons there is a strong argument for persuading parents to prevent children with grommets from swimming in chlorinated water, although perhaps a less valid one against swimming in the sea, provided the children keep to the surface.

Acute mastoiditis

Mastoiditis arises only when there is breakdown of the thin bony partition between the mastoid air cells – a process which takes two to three weeks (Figure 3.6). During that time, from the onset of

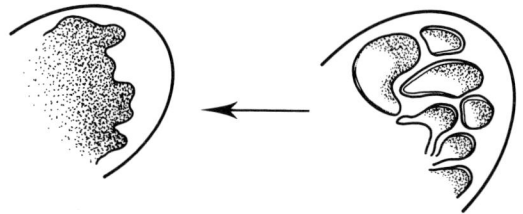

Figure 3.6 Acute mastoiditis.

an acute otitis media, there is continuing and increasingly copious discharge through a perforation in the drum. If a patient has pain a few days after the drum has been reliably shown to be normal, then he cannot have developed mastoiditis. Difficulties in diagnosis arise when an acute otitis media is thought to have recovered but has in fact grumbled on. Sometimes, because of systemic antibiotics, this may have been associated with very little systemic disturbance. Mastoiditis must be suspected in any patient with continuous discharge from the middle ear for over ten days, particularly if there is general malaise.

A patient in these circumstances should be referred for otological examination. Radiographs of the mastoid may help but not always. Only if a clearly aerated normal cell system is shown can mastoiditis be excluded. A classical appearance of breakdown of intracellular trabeculae is not always visible. Otitis externa, with oedema of soft tissue over the mastoid, may cause haziness of the cell system. The classical swelling behind the ear, which causes downward displacement of the pinna, implies a subperiosteal abscess, and this is a complication rather than a feature of mastoiditis. A subperiosteal abscess (Figure 3.7) can, by *erosion of the outer attic wall,* cause swelling in the *deep part* of the ear canal; this should be contrasted with a furuncle, which arises only in the outer part. If doubt remains about possible mastoiditis, the otologist will elect to explore the mastoid region under anaesthetic.

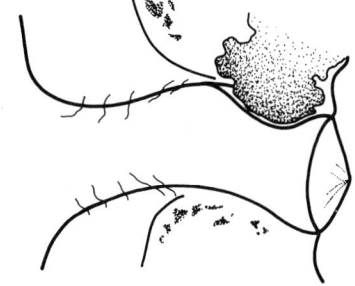

Figure 3.7 A subperiosteal abscess.

Ear pain without signs of inflammatory disease

Referred pain from outside the ear is the most likely explanation, either from disease in the oropharynx (IXth nerve), the laryngopharynx (Xth nerve), the upper molar teeth, the parotid gland, the temporomandibular joint (Vth nerve, mandibular division), or the cervical spine (C2 and C3) (Figure 3.8). If referred pain is suspected, the need for a full otolaryngological examination will necessitate referral to an ENT outpatient department.

Finally, rare causes of pain in the ear to be considered if none of the above have been found include tympanic (glossopharyngeal) neuralgia, migrainous neuralgia, and psychological disorders such as depression.

18 Ear, nose and throat conditions

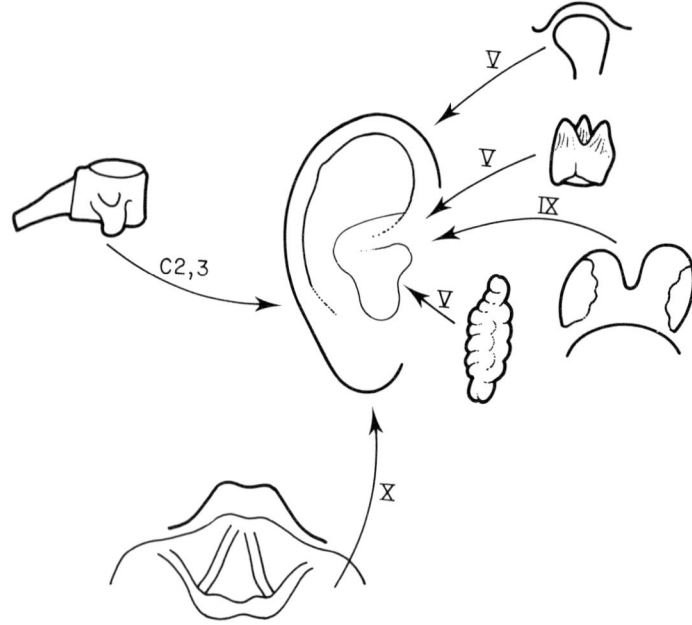

Figure 3.8 Pain referred to the ear.

Chronic suppurative otitis media

This name is applied to disorders with long-standing discharge through a tympanic membrane perforation, usually without pain. There is a conductive deafness. Two varieties are recognized – the safe and the unsafe.

The safe variety
This entails no risk of intracranial or life-threatening complications. The disease affects the mucosa of the lower anterior or tubotympanic part of the middle-ear cleft (Figure 3.9). It goes through stages of activity when the mucosa discharges through the perforation in the ear-drum, and periods of quiescence when the ear is dry and the patient is affected purely by the previous damage to the drum and middle-ear structures.

The unsafe variety
By contrast, the unsafe variety affects the atticoantral part of the middle ear (Figure 3.10) and threatens serious complications such as facial paralysis, sigmoid sinus thrombophlebitis, suppurative labyrinthitis, meningitis, subdural abscess, and brain abcess. The disease is dangerous because it is associated with bone

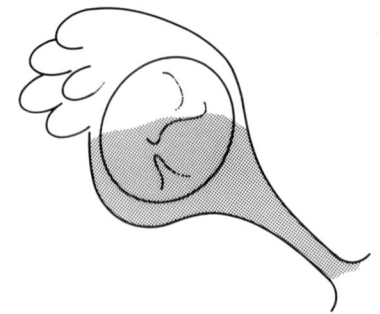

Figure 3.9 Chronic suppurative otitis media (safe variety).

erosion by cholesteatoma and by chronic osteitis in the affected regions.

In the safe type the *perforation* in the ear-drum is central, which is to say that there is always a rim of drum, or its annulus, around the edge (Figure 3.11). In contrast, the perforation in the unsafe type extends to the very bony edge of the drum and is called 'marginal' (Figure 3.12). A marginal perforation usually affects the posterior part of the ear-drum or the attic, and this characteristic reflects the pathological way in which

Ear diseases 19

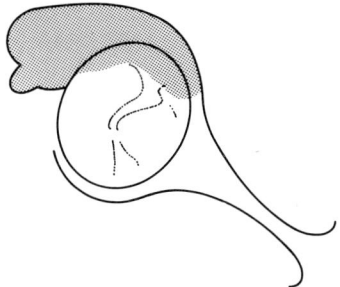

Figure 3.10 Chronic suppurative otitis media (unsafe variety).

cholesteatoma has developed from the skin of the ear-drum by invagination into the middle-ear cleft. The discharge in the safe variety is mucoid and intermittent, often provoked by blockage of the Eustachian tube and by upper respiratory tract infections, or by water passing into the middle ear through the perforation. The discharge from the unsafe variety is usually scanty and foul smelling, and there are no periods of quiescence. This discharge arises from the infected debris accumulating within the cholesteatoma sac.

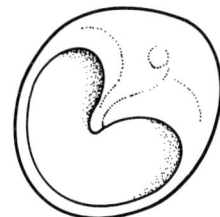

Figure 3.11 Central perforation.

The recognition of the disorder involves careful examination of the ear after removing discharge and debris. This may not be feasible in general practice, and any patients with chronic discharge should be referred to an ENT department where the ear can be examined under an operating microscope. It will then also be possible to carry out tuning-fork tests and audiometric tests to identify the presence and severity of any conductive deafnesss. It is often necessary to examine the ears on more than one occasion before being able safely to establish the nature of a chronic middle-ear disease.

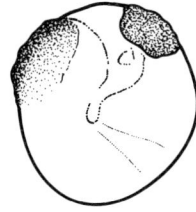

Figure 3.12 Marginal perforations.

Facial palsy and vertigo
These are both symptoms of complications of chronic middle-ear disease, and it is essential that the ears of any patient with these disorders be competently examined. If, as is often the case, it is not possible to see the whole tympanic membrane with an otoscope because of debris or wax scabs, then removal of these under a microscope in the outpatient department may be necessary. In rare instances examination of the ear under a general anaesthetic is advisable to exclude the possibility of dangerous middle-ear disease.

Treatment
In managing chronic middle-ear disease there is *no place for the use of systemic antibiotics*. The commonest organisms, which are Gram-negative commensals, are not sensitive to any of the safe systemic antibiotics, and their proliferation in an avascular region renders them inaccessible to such drugs. In both forms of chronic middle-ear disease there is a useful place for the application of topical antibiotic and steroid drops to control infection and reduce inflammatory reaction. Any drugs administered should be warmed to body temperature by holding the bottle under a hot tap, and massaged into the middle ear (Figure 3.13).

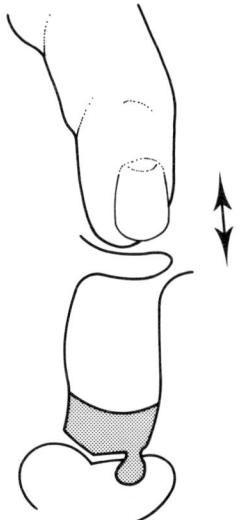

Figure 3.13 Administration of topical drugs.

With a safe infection this treatment, if done regularly, may be sufficient to eliminate the discharge and render the ear dry, while with the unsafe variety such topical application, used for a week or two, will provide conditions for a better outpatient assessment of the state of the ear. Ultimately the management of every unsafe variety of ear infection involves surgical operation.

Operations to be considered

These are radical mastoidectomy, modified radical mastoidectomy, atticotomy, and atticoantrostomy. In all, the aim is to remove diseased and infected bone and to leave a smooth, wide cavity opening into a wide external ear canal. As the ear heals that cavity becomes lined with skin. Although this will be histologically identical to cholesteatoma, it will be able to excrete its dead squames to the exterior through wide access.

Mastoidectomy A radical mastoidectomy operation leaves the patient with a mastoid cavity communicating with the external ear canal (Figure 3.14), which will require regular outpatient attention. Eighty per cent of such cavities become dry, with a clean skin lining, and these require the removal of wax once a year indefinitely. If for any reason the skin fails to line the whole cavity, the ear will continue to discharge; in some ears the skin lining is intermittently unstable, breaking down when affected by water from outside, so that patches of denuded lining exude a discharge. During such periods the application of antibiotic or steroid drops may rapidly produce a dry cavity again. As in the management of chronic otitis media, there is no merit in prescribing systemic antibiotics to a patient with a discharging mastoidectomy cavity.

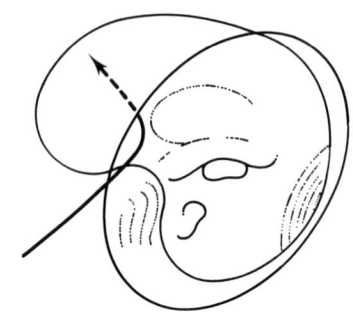

Figure 3.14 Mastoidectomy.

Deafness

There are two forms of deafness:
1. That due to defects in *conduction* caused by perforation in the ear drum, loss of continuity of the ossicular chain, fixation of the ossicular chain, obstruction of the Eustachian tube, and of course obstruction of the external ear canal (Figure 3.15).
2. That due to deficiencies in *sensorineural mechanisms* caused for instance by degenerative age changes, noise exposure, ototoxic drugs, Menière's disease, and acoustic neuroma.

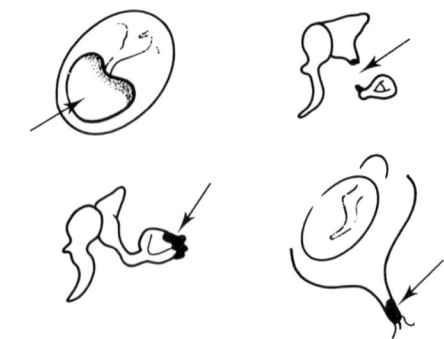

Figure 3.15 Defects in conduction.

Conductive hearing loss

Glue ear is treated surgically by the insertion of a ventilation tube or grommet.
Otosclerosis may be helped by stapedectomy to replace the fixed stapes with a mobile prosthesis.
A perforated drum can be repaired by a myringoplasty grafting operation.

Ossicular defects may be corrected surgically by reconstruction of the ossicular chain (ossiculoplasty or tympanoplasty).

When considering possible operation, the risk of damaging inner-ear function must be considered. This is as high as 2 per cent in stapedectomy operations, despite an overall success rate of 90 per cent. The risk is much lower in myringoplasty, with a graft success rate of about 90 per cent, and is negligible for grommet insertion.

If operation is not advisable, a hearing aid should be tried with any hard-of-hearing patient.

Sudden sensorineural hearing loss

Sudden loss of hearing, fortunately, usually affects only one ear, but it should constitute a medical emergency. Any patient who has suddenly (over the course of a few days) suffered a severe hearing loss in one ear should be referred for otological investigation. There are many possible causes which will have to be excluded by investigation. *In the majority of cases no cause will be identified.*

Acoustic neuromas not infrequently present with this syndrome.

Viral infections probably can cause sudden sensorineural hearing loss; certainly the virus of herpes zoster oticus has been implicated, as has that of mumps.

Traumatic tears of intralabyrinthine membranes (Figure 3.16), with leakage of perilymph from the oval window or round window into the middle ear, may be preceded by trauma of very slight degree, such as slight exertion or mild closed-head injury.

Syphilitic infection of the temporal bone is another possible cause.

Investigation
Investigation of such patients then will involve assessment of the hearing defect, assessment of vestibular function, specific serological tests, x-rays and tomograms of the internal auditory meatuses, and in some instances more elaborate procedures to exclude acoustic neuroma.

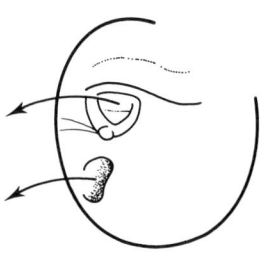

Figure 3.16 Tears of intralabyrinthine membranes.

Management
This should take place in hospital. If a perilymph leak is suspected the patient will be nursed sitting up. Empirical treatment will usually involve the use of systemic steroids in large doses and vasodilator drugs to increase cochlear blood flow, although it must be admitted that there is no strong proof that these measures have any effect on the outcome. Operative exploration of the middle ear will be considered to seal any perilymph leak.

Unilateral sensorineural hearing loss

Whether of sudden onset or not, any patient with a unilateral sensorineural hearing loss must be considered to have a *possible acoustic neuroma*. These tumours arise from the Schwann cells, usually of the superior vestibular nerve, in the internal auditory meatus, and present with hearing loss, tinnitus, and vague instability. Severe vertigo is very rare. The hearing loss, as has been mentioned, may be of sudden onset but is more usually slow, insidious, and progressive. In 98 per cent of instances the tumour is unilateral. It expands within the internal auditory meatus (Figure 3.17) and then spreads into the cerebellopontine angle where it produces symptoms affecting the Vth nerve, with numbness of the face,

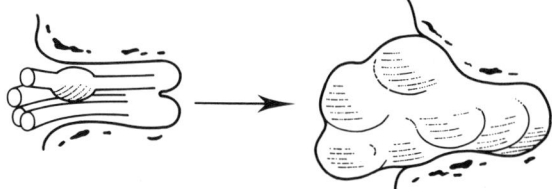

Figure 3.17 Acoustic neuroma.

and eventually compression of the brain stem with ataxia, and central vestibular disturbances. In the final stages the tumour will cause raised intracranial pressure with papilloedema and finally death.

The suspicion of an acoustic neuroma requires referral to an otology department, where appropriate investigations can be conducted. *Audiometric tests* will help to distinguish between a fault in the cochlea and one of the auditory nerve, and specialized hearing tests by brain-stem evoked-response audiometry are highly sensitive. *X-rays* and tomograms of the internal auditory meatuses will be necessary; and if these are abnormal, with enlargement and possible bone erosion around the meatus on the suspected side, *high-resolution computerized tomogram scanning* will be advised. Unfortunately CT scanning cannot demonstrate tumours smaller than about 1½ cm in diameter, and in these circumstances, if suspicion remains high, contrast metography will be necessary. This involves the instillation of some contrast medium, usually gas or air, into the internal auditory meatus during the performance of a high-resolution CT scan. Although investigation along these lines is necessary in any patient with unilateral sensorineural hearing loss and in many patients with unilateral tinnitus, a relatively small percentage of patients investigated will be found to have tumours. Nonetheless, early recognition of tumours facilitates their removal with much less risk to the facial nerve, and much lower morbidity, than when a large tumour needs to be excised. Postoperative problems include the almost inevitable loss of hearing, and the management of facial paralysis which may later be helped by faciohypoglossal anastomosis.

Vertigo

By definition vertigo is an illusion of movement and should not be taken merely as a synonym for imbalance. Balance will be impaired by defects in sensory information from the eyes, proprioceptive receptors, and the vestibular labyrinth, by defects in accurate co-ordination of sensory information within the brain, and by faults in the functioning motor output from the central nervous system to the normal musculoskeletal system (Figure 3.18). Vertigo occurs when information from vestibular sources conflicts with that from other sensory systems, or when a disordered central integrating system does not coherently assess the body's movements from vestibular information. Vertigo, then, is always a symptom of vestibular defect, whether it lies in the peripheral labyrinth or in its connections within the brain. When severe it is usually accompanied by nausea and vomiting.

Vertigo can be caused by (a) peripheral vestibular (labyrinthine) disorders, (b) central vestibular disorders such as multiple sclerosis, tumours, or infarcts, and (c) external influences on the vestibular system by drugs, anaemia, hypoglycaemia, hypotension, viral infection, and,

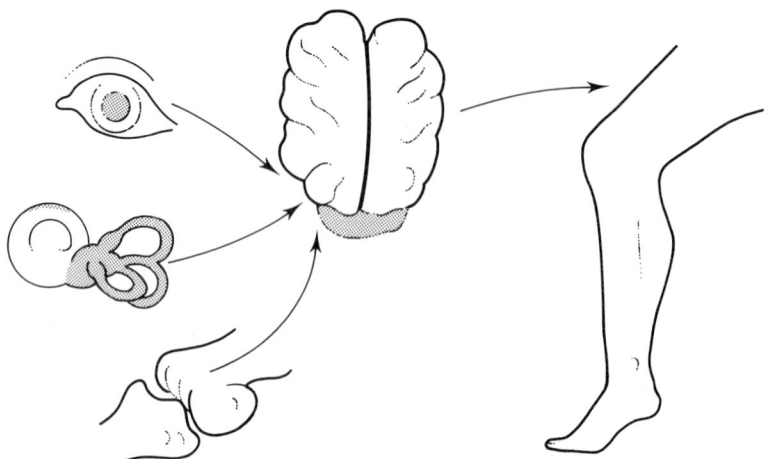

Figure 3.18 Factors affecting balance.

most important, by erosion of the bony walls of the labyrinth by destructive middle-ear disease.

The commonest peripheral vestibular disorders are:

benign paroxysmal positional vertigo
Menière's disease and other forms of endolymphatic hydrops
sudden vestibular failure
vascular disturbances.

These account for over 75 per cent of cases of vertigo.

Benign paroxysmal positional vertigo

This is the commonest cause of paroxysmal vertigo and the diagnosis is often overlooked because of failure to perform a positional test. It is provoked by movements of the head, usually to one side when turning in bed or looking upwards. An attack lasts for a few seconds and there are no auditory symptoms. The disorder is due to 'cupulolithiasis' in which calcium carbonate crystals from the otoconia of the otolith organ in an affected utricle become detached. They fall against the cupula of the posterior semicircular canal. The underlying cause may be viral infection, degenerative changes, or trauma. Usually the cause is uncertain. The history is suggestive, and the diagnosis can be made simply by *positional testing*. The patient is seated on a couch, head towards the examiner, and is told to watch the examiner's forehead. The observer, holding the patient's head, rapidly lays him back into a supine position with his head over the edge of the couch – 30° below the horizontal (Figure 3.19). He is held there for at least 30 seconds, during which time the observer watches the patient's eyes for nystagmus. The test is then repeated with the head turned to the other side. Nystagmus provoked by this test is always abnormal. Positional nystagmus is found in benign positional vertigo but it can also, rarely, indicate a vestibular lesion in the posterior cranial fossa. In benign paroxysmal positional vertigo, the nystagmus invariably shows the following features: (a) there is a latent period of some seconds before its onset, (b) it abates after 5 to 20 seconds in the provoking position and is less violent on repeated testing, (c) it is always rotatory, beating towards the underlying ear, (d) it is always accompanied by violent vertigo, (e) it does not change direction during observation. Lack of any of those features should suggest a central cause for the positional nystagmus.

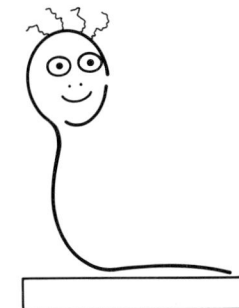

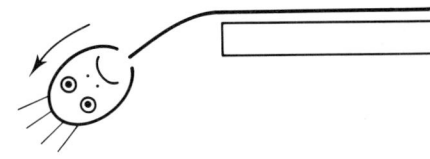

Figure 3.19 Positional testing.

Management of benign positional vertigo

There is no specific treatment apart from avoidance of the provoking head positions. Vestibular sedatives rarely help. Some patients suffer repeated bouts of the condition, but most recover within a few weeks and are then free from trouble. Under the very rare circumstances of prolonged repeated attacks, vestibular head exercises may be advised to try to retrain the brain to accept the abnormal impulse. As a last resort the nerve to the posterior semicircular canal ampulla can be surgically sectioned.

Sudden vestibular failure

This presents an entirely different time pattern from the previous disorder. It arises when one peripheral labyrinth suddenly stops working. That may be for various reasons, including closed head injuries, viral infections (such as varicella zoster), blockage of an end artery to the labyrinth, brain-stem encephalitis, and multiple sclerosis. The effects of the disorder are the onset of sudden vertigo with prostration, nausea and vomiting. There are no auditory symptoms, and unlike the previous condition the vertigo persists continuously, gradually abating over many days or weeks. It is exacerbated by head movements, but after a few days it may lessen unless the head is turned suddenly. A young, healthy patient gradually regains full balance by the end of ten days or so as a result of compensation in processes taking place within the brain. Recovery is much less complete and slower in old age, and imbalance may return temporarily at any time, whenever the acquired compensation breaks down as a result of defects in other sensory systems – other illnesses, fatigue, drugs, or cerebral degeneration.

Investigation
The history is characteristic. As with the other forms of vertigo it is essential that the ears be carefully examined to exclude chronic middle-ear disease. In sudden vestibular failure there will be seen a third-degree jerk nystagmus towards the unaffected ear, and as the days pass that will gradually subside to a second-degree, then a first-degree state, and will finally disappear (Figure 3.20), although special investigations will still show the jerk nystagmus when the eyes are examined in darkness.

idiopathic. The condition usually affects only one ear with the first symptoms between the ages of 30 and 60 years. It is characterized by attacks of violent paroxysmal vertigo which is usually rotatory, associated with deafness and tinnitus. The attacks occur in clusters with periods of remission. An individual attack lasts for several hours, and Menière's disease should not lightly be diagnosed when the vertigo lasts for less than ten minutes or more than 12 hours. There is generally prostration, nausea and vomiting and often a sensation of pressure in the ear, and an increase or change in the character of the tinnitus. Menière's disease does not cause loss of consciousness.

The accompanying deafness is sensorineural and fluctuates in severity. *Fluctuating hearing loss* is caused more frequently by hydrops of the endolymphatic system than by Eustachian-tube obstruction. This fluctuating hearing defect may develop before the first attack of vertigo. Between attacks the hearing tends to improve, but over a period of time it deteriorates until the loss has become severe. Tinnitus is low pitched or roaring and varies with the hearing level. In 60 to 70 per cent of patients with Menière's disease one ear only is affected. In the remainder with bilateral

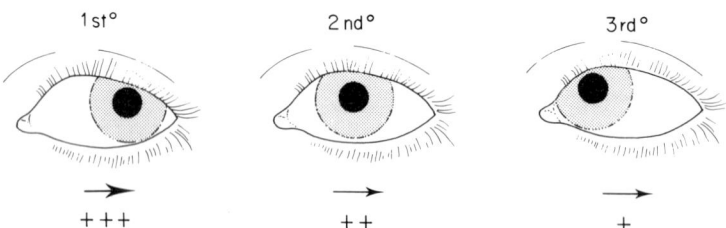

Figure 3.20 Degrees of jerk nystagmus.

Management
In severe cases, during the first few days the patient should be kept in bed and given vestibular sedatives either by injection or as suppositories. After the first few days, oral medication with the same drugs may be continued.

Menière's disease

This is a disorder of endolymph control with dilatation of endolymphatic spaces of the membranous labyrinth. Such dilatation, or hydrops, may be caused by disorders of the otic capsule such as Paget's disease and labyrinthine syphilis, but by definition, in Menière's disease it is

disease the deafness may become more severe than the vertigo, and after many years of activity the imbalance suffered by the patient may not be due to vertigo but to deficit of the vestibular system on each side. Menière-like episodic vertigo without auditory symptoms can arise from hydrops affecting only the vestibular part of the labyrinth.

Diagnosis
The diagnosis can usually be made from the history. It is commonly over-diagnosed by associating tinnitus from other causes, such as presbyacusis, with unsteadiness for other reasons, say old-age degenerative changes or brain-stem ischaemia. Full diagnosis requires referral to

hospital for audiometric tests to identify the characteristic kind of hearing defect, or for investigations described above to exclude an acoustic neuroma, and for appropriate investigations to exclude other possible causes such as Paget's disease.

Management

During an acute attack the vertigo can be helped by the administration of prochlorperazine or cinnarizine either by injection or as a suppository. Between attacks vertigo may be suppressed by the oral use of the same drugs. Vasodilator drugs such as betahistine (Serc), 8 mg three times daily, to increase cochlear blood flow may help. In some patients fluid balance factors seem to play a part, and restriction of salt intake combined with the administration of diuretics, such as frusemide or hydrochlorothiazide may be helpful.

Surgical treatment will be considered whenever a patient with severe symptoms fails to respond to a few months' medical care. There are many options, but if the hearing is good the operation of *endolymphatic sac decompression* will produce relief from vertigo in 85 per cent or more of patients. If the hearing is very poor then total destruction of the labyrinth by labyrinthectomy may be advisable (Figure 3.21), although there will always be anxiety about the hearing in the other ear. Vestibular nerve section (Figure 3.22) has a place for the small number of patients with good hearing who have not been helped by saccus decompression surgery.

Any patient in whom there is doubt about diagnosis, and any who has not responded to medical treatment after six weeks should be referred for otological investigation and advice.

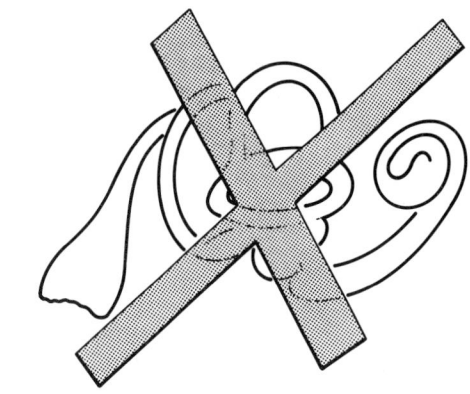

Figure 3.21 Labyrinthectomy.

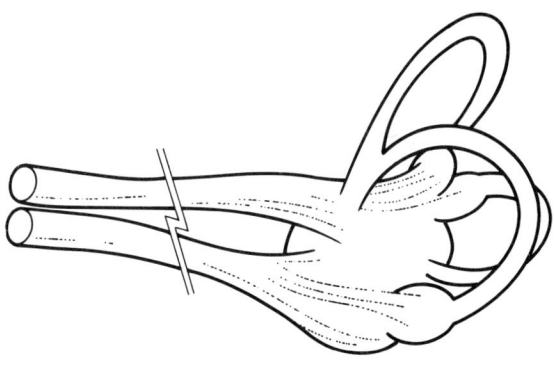

Figure 3.22 Vestibular nerve section.

Facial palsy

Lower motor neurone facial palsies are usually idiopathic, but that label can be attached only after full investigations and exclusion of other possible causes.

These other causes include:

Intracranial lesions such as neoplasms, multiple sclerosis, cerebellopontine-angle masses, and poliomyelitis.

Intratemporal causes, including trauma by ear surgery or head injury, otitis media (especially chronic with cholesteatoma), herpes zoster oticus (Ramsay Hunt syndrome), and rarely carcinoma of the middle ear or neuromas of the facial nerve.

Extracranial conditions, including trauma or carcinoma of the parotid gland.

Other rare causes, including sarcoidosis, infections mononucleosis, and polyneuritis.

Full diagnosis
This involves identification of the site of the lesion, recognition of the cause, and assessment of the severity of the involvement of the nerve. Only when these three characteristics have been defined can a facial palsy be correctly described, rational treatment planned, and a reliable prognosis given.

Clinical assessment
Clinical assessment involves examination of movement of each part of the face during voluntary and emotional movement. Sparing of the forehead and paralysis of voluntary rather than involuntary movement suggests an upper motor neurone lesion.

As with vertigo, careful examination of the tympanic membranes is essential. Cholesteatoma may be hidden by a crust over the outer attic wall and this may be overlooked (Figure 3.23). If suspected the ear must be examined under an operating microscope, and for diagnostic purposes the middle ear must on occasions be opened surgically. Examination of the pinna and the ear canal may reveal the rash and blisters typical of the Ramsay Hunt syndrome. Assessment of the

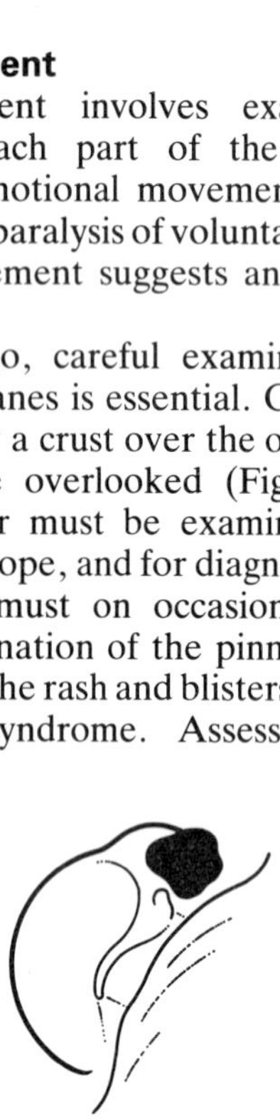

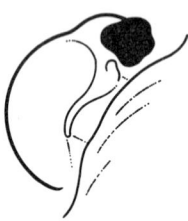

Figure 3.23 Cholesteatoma.

integrity of branches of the facial nerve, helpful in identifying the site of the lesion, requires examination of lacrimation and taste. Lacrimation is examined by *Schirmer's test*. A strip of sterile filter paper is folded at one end and hung on to each lower eyelid (Figure 3.24). The rate of moistening of the papers as tears run along them is compared between the two sides. Taste from the anterior two-thirds of the tongue is more difficult to test, and the patient's observations about disturbance of taste at the time of onset are often valuable. If at this stage of examination the cause of paralysis does not become apparent, the patient should be referred for radiological examination of the temporal bone.

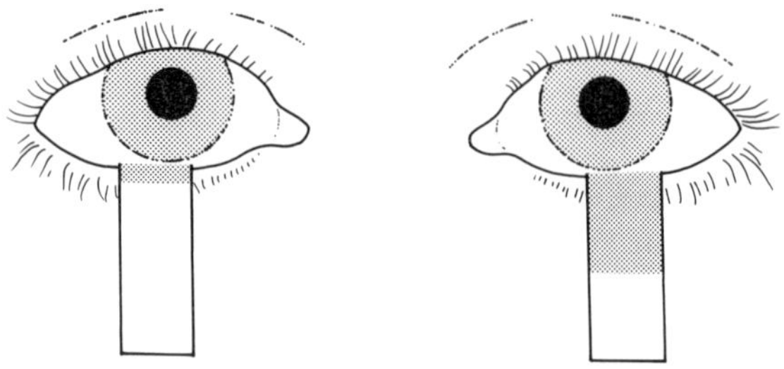

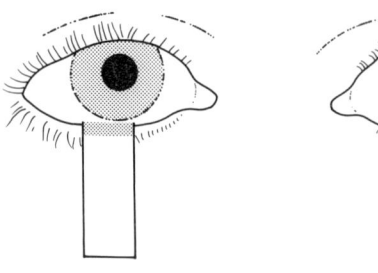

Figure 3.24 Schirmer's test.

The site of the lesion
This is determined by the following considerations. The great superficial petrosal nerve arises from the geniculate ganglion in the petrous temporal bone, and carries fibres destined to innervate the lacrimal gland (Figure 3.25). Just before leaving the temporal bone (above the stylomastoid foramen) the facial nerve is joined by the chorda tympani carrying sensory taste fibres from the anterior two-thirds of the tongue. A short way above, a small branch supplies motor fibres to the stapedius muscle. From this anatomical structure it follows that a lesion in the brain produces weakness only of the facial muscles with no loss of taste or lacrimation. There are often other neurological signs. Loss of lacrimation and of taste from the anterior two-thirds of the tongue indicate a lesion between the brain stem and the geniculate ganglion. If the facial weakness is associated with loss of taste, but with sparing of lacrimation, the inference must be that the lesion lies between the geniculate ganglion and the origin of the chorda tympani. Preservation of both taste and lacrimation are to be expected when the lesion is peripheral to the stylomastoid foramen, and in these circumstances of course no other cranial nerve defects will usually be apparent. Affection of the nerve by injury or by disease is usually apparent from a consideration of the history or the clinical examination. More rarely surgical exploration of the nerve may be needed in order to establish the diagnosis. In most cases, however, if the facial paralysis has been of sudden onset and there is no apparent explanation on clinical or x-ray examination, it may be described as a Bell's palsy.

Facial palsy

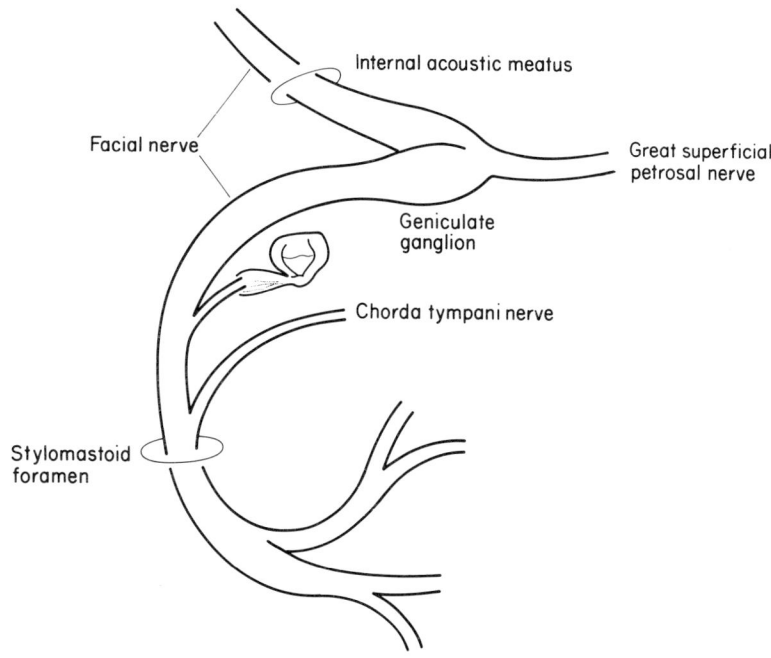

Figure 3.25 Facial nerve and geniculate ganglion.

Severity of the lesion

It is important to know whether the nerve has suffered damage (neurotmesis or axonotmesis) from which it can recover only by regeneration, or whether the damage is slighter (neurapraxia), from which it may recover rapidly without degeneration taking place. This assessment of severity is usually made by electrodiagnostic tests. Neurapraxia may be assumed whenever movement is retained in all divisions of the nerve. Whenever a nerve is damaged, for example by injury or division, no electrical test can demonstrate abnormality until the peripheral part of the nerve has degenerated as far as the region where the test stimulus is applied. This distal degeneration takes from *three to five days* to reach the stylomastoid foramen, at which point nerve conduction tests are performed (Figure 3.26). It follows then that no electrical test can demonstrate degeneration until this interval after the onset of facial paralysis. Conversely if electrical tests are normal one week after the onset of the paralysis it may confidently be assumed that degeneration has not occurred, even though the face is totally paralysed.

Treatment

Early treatment

In facial palsy this has to deal with any causative lesion, to alleviate any disability, and to offer the nerve the best chances of recovery. Treatment of the causative lesion may involve, for example, operative treatment of chronic middle-ear disease, surgical removal of a tumour involving the facial nerve, or whatever else may be appropriate. In relieving the disability, the cornea of the affected side must be protected. An eye cover or a wing to a spectacle frame may be adequate for a short period, but if recovery is expected to take many months a lateral partial tarsorrhaphy should be carried out. The appearance of the face may be improved by lifting the corner of the mouth with a device called a 'plumper', attached by a dental surgeon to an upper plate or to existing teeth. There is no evidence that massage or electrical stimulation of the paralysed muscle either prevents atrophy or encourages recovery.

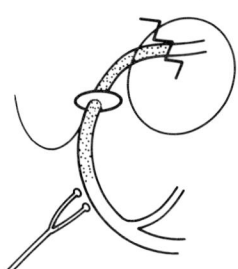

Figure 3.26 Nerve degeneration.

Help for the nerve depends on whether the fibres are in continuity, or whether they have been severed and the ends separated. If voluntary movement persists, or if electrical responses remain normal for a long period, continuity of the nerve may be assumed. If total degeneration is indicated by electrical tests, and there is doubt about the possible continuity, as may be the case after trauma, surgical exploration is often necessary to determine the state of the nerve. At operation breaches of continuity may be repaired by inserting nerve grafts taken from the sural nerve in the leg (Figure 3.27).

Late treatment
In those patients who have suffered facial paralysis without recovery after a year, an anastomosis between the hypoglossal nerve and the facial nerve (Figure 3.28) will produce good movement of the face, and is preferable to alternative measures such as plastic surgery to raise the paralysed side of the face with a facial sling. Two to three years after the onset of the facial paralysis the facial muscles will have undergone atrophy and plastic surgery alone will be helpful.

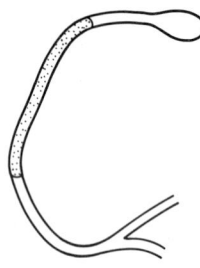

Figure 3.27 Nerve graft.

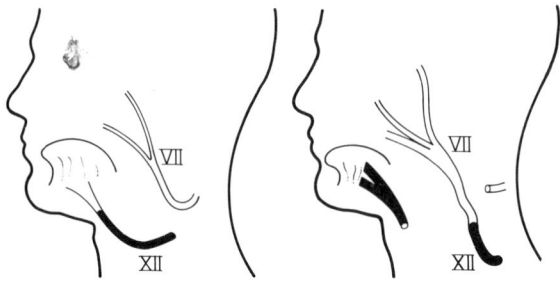

Figure 3.28 Facio-hypoglossal anastomosis.

Although the cause of Bell's palsy is uncertain there is some evidence that systemic steroids are useful, and they may be advocated in all patients who do not have contraindications to their use – such as hypertension, pregnancy, diabetes, peptic ulceration or pulmonary tuberculosis. Prednisolone, 20 mg four times a day should be given for five days and then tailed off over a further five days. In a Bell's palsy with total degeneration of the nerve there is occasionally a case for surgical decompression of the nerve to allow the oedematous contents within the nerve sheath to expand.

Prognosis
This depends on whether the nerve has degenerated. If neurapraxia alone has taken place recovery will always be complete provided the cause is controlled. When degeneration has taken place recovery will occur by regeneration provided the nerve is in continuity, but this will take several months and there will be only partial recovery marred by associated movements, involuntary clonic twitching, and contractures. In Bell's palsy 90 per cent or more of patients recover fully.

Nasal problems

Symptoms referred to the nose most often affect children, young adults, and the middle-aged.

The nose is constantly exposed to inhaled irritants, allergens, pollutants and pathogens – hence it is scarcely surprising that it suffers and reacts.

Nasal obstruction

In childhood Chronic nasal obstruction is caused most frequently by vasomotor rhinitis or by adenoid enlargement. Much rarer causes are congenital choanal atresia, and tumours of the postnasal space.

In adult life Nasal obstruction is caused most commonly by vasomotor rhinitis or by a deflection of the nasal septum, and somewhat less commonly by the mucosal swelling and redundancies associated with vasomotor rhinitis such as ethmoid polyps and 'moriform' fringes on the turbinates.

Chronic sinusitis is nowadays a very rare cause of nasal obstruction.

Even more rare are *benign and malignant tumours* of the nose, the paranasal sinuses and the nasopharynx, and *granulomatous diseases* caused by bacterial infections such as tuberculosis, syphilis and leprosy.

Of importance is *iatrogenic nasal obstruction* from the excessive use of topical vasoconstrictors – rhinitis medicamentosa.

Occasional nasal obstruction of course is very common, and people vary greatly in their tolerance of a blocked nose. Some with normal nasal patency complain of persisting nasal obstruction, while others with an obviously blocked nose make no complaint.

Vasomotor rhinitis

This is the commonest cause of persisting nasal obstruction in children and adults. It is a disorder of the normal control of swelling and shrinking of the nasal mucosa, necessary for its air-conditioning function. There may be external allergic causes. The condition will be seasonal when allergens such as grass pollen appear for short periods at the same time each year, or perennial in the presence of allergens such as the house-dust mite (*Dermatophagoides*). In children allergic vasomotor rhinitis is often associated with a family history of atopy, and with eczema and allergic asthma. Sneezing and rhinorrhoea are as troublesome as nasal obstruction. Often there is no recognizable allergen, and there may be external irritating causes in the form of changes in temperature and humidity; or chemical irritants to which the nasal mucosa is unduly sensitive. Intrinsic factors such as hormonal changes and emotional disturbances may also be relevant.

Persisting perennial nasal obstruction

When due to vasomotor rhinitis this is often associated with oedema of the nasal mucosa, producing redundant folds and lumps. These can take the form of ethmoid polyps, antrochoanal polyps, or swellings and fringes on the turbinates (Figure 3.29). Ethmoid nasal polyps are swellings arising from the lining of the ethmoid air cells which protrude into the nose. Constriction at the ostium of the air cells increases the oedema within the polyps so that they expand within the nasal

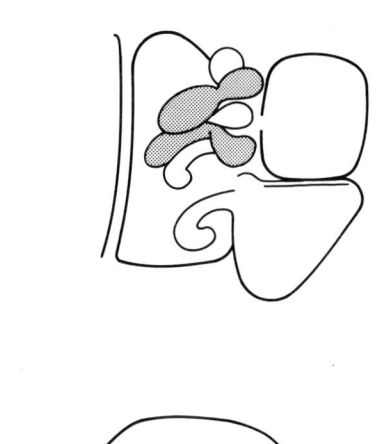

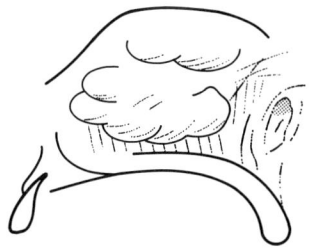

Figure 3.29 Nasal obstruction.

cavity. Antrochoanal polyps are much rarer, and arise from the maxillary antrum, passing through its ostium backwards to the posterior choana. They tend to be commoner in children and adolescents than in adults, because of the smaller size of the antrum. Swellings, or moriform fringes, along the edges of the inferior turbinates are often found in the noses of patients with persisting vasomotor rhinitis.

Rhinitis medicamentosa

This can follow the use of any nasal decongestant spray. It seems probable that the mucosa is damaged by the severe vasoconstriction causing anoxia. Each episode of decongestion is followed by a rebound engorgement of the nasal mucosa, which encourages the patient to apply the spray again. The inevitable effect of such sprays is potential addiction, so they should be used only when the underlying condition is likely to abate within a week or so.

Blocked nose in childhood

A history will give some indication of the degree of disturbance caused by the obstruction. A detailed account of the history during sleep is important. It is now becoming increasingly recognized that some children suffer periods of apnoea and hypoxia at night. This sort of obstructive apnoea, which is sometimes caused by enlarged adenoids and tonsils, may be responsible for a failure to thrive, for sleep deprivation, for deformitites of the chest, and much more rarely for serious cardiovascular disturbances such as cor pulmonale.

When examining a child who has an open-mouthed posture it is necessary to decide if the child is still breathing through the nose despite the open mouth, as is often the case. Holding a cold, shiny speculum under the nose and observing condensation during expiration is one way of detecting nasal breathing (Figure 3.30). If only one side of the nose appears completely blocked the possibility of a unilateral posterior choanal atresia has to be considered. Examination of the front of the nose will often show the swollen mucosa expected in vasomotor rhinitis. This is often pale mauve in colour and the swelling of the anterior ends of the inferior turbinates is often mistakenly diagnosed as a nasal polyp.

Further investigation of childhood nasal obstruction might involve referral for a lateral soft-tissue x-ray of the postnasal space to show the degree of adenoid enlargement.

If the nasal obstruction interferes with sleep, causing apnoea or severe snoring, or affects speech, then referral to the ENT Department is advised.

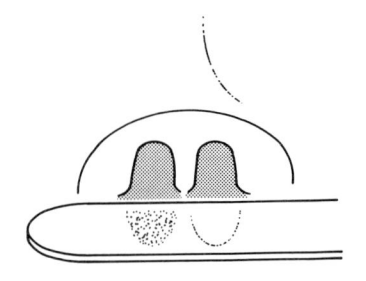

Figure 3.30 Detection of nasal breathing.

The surgical help available includes adenoidectomy, submucous diathermy of the swollen parts of the mucosa over the inferior turbinates in vasomotor rhinitis, or the appropriate surgical treatment for the rarer abnormalities causing nasal obstruction. Submucous diathermy involves a general anaesthetic and the application of diathermy current through a needle to tissues under the mucosa over the inferior turbinate (Figure 3.31). The simple procedure is followed by scarring of the injured tissue, with retraction of the swollen mucosa on to the turbinate bone. The benefits of the procedure usually last for several years, which may be a sufficiently long period to allow the interior of the nose to grow to a size when the oedematous mucosa can be accommodated.

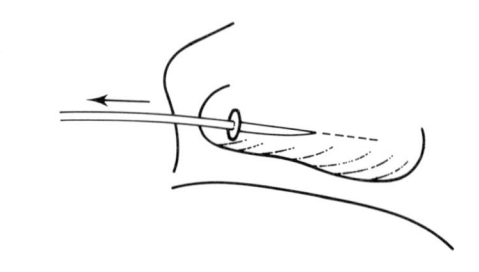

Figure 3.31 Submucous diathermy.

Nasal obstruction in the adult

Although the history is important, the assessment depends mainly on examination of the postnasal space with a mirror, and of the anterior nares with a Thudichum speculum. Response of the mucosa to a vasoconstrictor spray can be very useful.

As with a child, if nasal obstruction is due to

some cause not treatable by simply medical means and causes discomfort, mouth breathing, gingivitis, hallitosis, snoring, or sleep apnoea, then referral to an ENT Department may be advisable.

When vasomotor rhinitis is the cause, submucous diathermy of the nasal mucosa may be as useful, as in childhood.

Ethmoid nasal polyps

Ethmoid polyps should be removed surgically, and in many instances the ethmoid cells from which the polyps arise should be exenterated, throwing each into continuity with its neighbour (Figure 3.32).

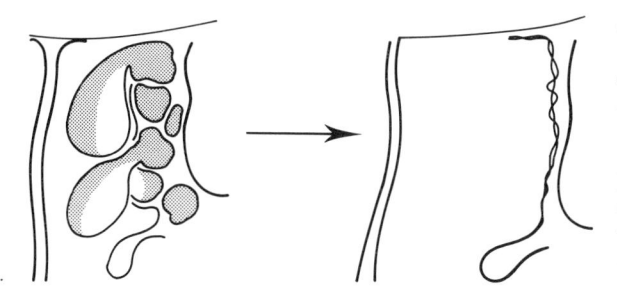

Figure 3.32 Ethmoidectomy.

This procedure of *ethmoidectomy* may be performed through the nose – intranasally – but in some instances, for more complete clearance with less risk of damage to surrounding structures, an external approach through an incision around the inner canthus of the eye may be used. Antrochoanal polyps are best treated by a Caldwell–Luc operation to open the maxillary antrum and remove all the oedematous mucosa from which the polyp has arisen. Swellings and moriform fringes on turbinate bones may be excised surgically.

A deviated nasal septum

This requires treatment only when it is the cause of troublesome nasal obstruction. In these circumstances a *submucous resection* operation is useful. The operation, which is usually performed under a general anaesthetic, involves 'filleting' the nasal septum by removing all the cartilage and bone which is holding the mucosal surfaces of the septum in the wrong position (Figure 3.33). The intact layers of mucosa left after this procedure come into contact with each other and hang in the midline. The operation carries a slight risk of perforation in the nasal septum, and an even smaller risk of collapse of the support of the nasal bridge with deformity of the nose.

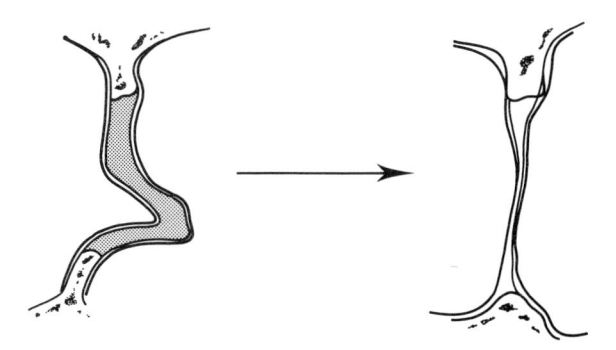

Figure 3.33 Submucous resection.

Chronic sinusitis

The condition is now uncommon in this country, but still much overdiagnosed. Bacterial infection arises when the self-cleansing mechanism of the paranasal sinuses is impaired. In those circumstances mucus accumulates and stagnates within the sinus cavities, and it becomes infected, usually by harmless opportunist bacteria found in the nose. The self-cleansing mechanism depends upon the continuity of a mucus blanket within the sinuses, swept by ciliary activity through their ostia into the nose. Thence the mucus is passed back into the nasopharynx and is swallowed. To work properly the mechanism requires secretion of mucus with the correct physical characteristics, normal function of the mucosal cilia, and patency of the ostia of the sinuses. Anatomical features place individual sinuses at different risk. The ostium of the maxillary antrum is high on its medial wall, so mucus has to be swept upwards against gravity. The frontal sinus has a long tortuous duct which is easily obstructed (Figure 3.34). The ethmoid cells open into the nose in regions where they may be bathed by infective material from the maxillary sinuses.

The commonest reason for derangement of self-cleansing is *viral infection of the nose and sinus mucosa*. This depresses activity of the cilia, and obstructs the sinus ostia by oedematous mucosa. Under these circumstances mucus accumulates in the paranasal sinuses on one or both sides. The process just described occurs whenever a patient is afflicted with an upper respiratory viral infection. Only if the self-cleansing mechanism does not recover will stagnating mucus become secondarily infected. The mucopus so produced impairs ciliary function and increases the circumostial swelling.

The main complaints in chronic sinusitis are of nasal obstruction and purulent nasal discharge.

Chronic maxillary sinusitis never causes swelling of the cheek. Headaches are frequently incorrectly ascribed to chronic sinusitis.

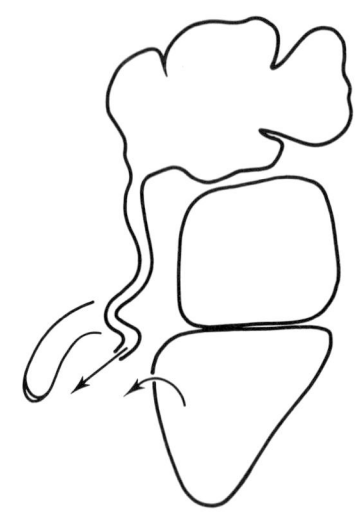

Figure 3.34 Frontal sinus duct.

Diagnosis

This may be suggested by clinical examination showing oedematous mucosa and mucopus in the nose or postnasal space, but a definitive diagnosis depends on the correct interpretation of sinus x-rays. Misinterpretation is a cause for overdiagnosis of chronic sinusitis. Loss of translucency in the maxillary sinuses may be due to mucosal swelling (Figure 3.35). This change is found in vasomotor

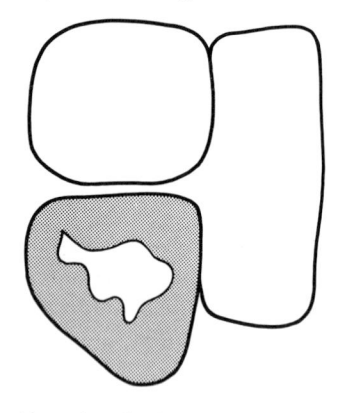

Figure 3.35 Mucosal swelling in maxillary sinus.

rhinitis, and during any acute upper respiratory tract viral infection — it does not indicate chronic sinus disease. It may be an ephemeral radiological appearance, and indeed sinus x-ray changes vary greatly from week to week. Chronic maxillary sinusitis can be suspected only if one or both antra are completely opaque – suggesting that they are filled with pus or mucopus and not simply with swollen mucosa, or if part of the sinus is completely opaque (Figure 3.36) with a fluid level at the air–liquid interface.

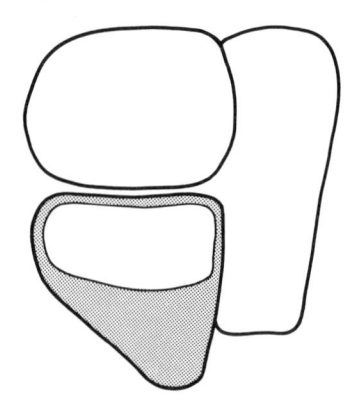

Figure 3.36 Fluid in maxillary sinus.

Treatment

The basis of treatment of chronic sinusitis is to break the vicious circle caused by the persistence of pus within a sinus cavity, in the hope of restoring normal self-cleansing.

Pus can be removed from the maxillary antrum by *washout*. This is a procedure performed under local anaesthesia in the adult, and involves the insertion of a hollow cannula through the nasal wall of the maxillary antrum under the inferior turbinate (Figure 3.37). Normal saline at body

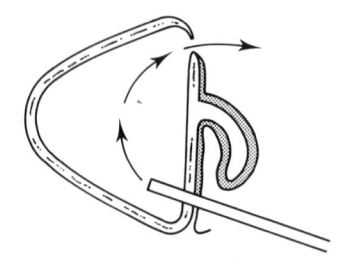

Figure 3.37 Pus washout.

temperature is irrigated through the antrum so that the contained pus escapes from the maxillary ostium into the nose, and pours into a bowl held under the patient's chin. This procedure may need to be repeated as an outpatient several times at weekly intervals. If self-cleansing recovers, the return from the washout will change from pus to clear fluid.

Failure of maxillary sinusitis to respond in this way is a reason for performing *intranasal antrostomy*. In this operation, carried out under a general anaesthetic, a ventilation hole is made from the maxillary sinus into the nose as low as possible below the inferior turbinate (Figure 3.38). This allows air entry and encourages the excretion of retained pus with recovery of the mucosa.

In rare instances the mucosa may be irreversibly diseased so that self-cleansing cannot recover. Under these circumstances a Caldwell–Luc operation is required. This involves an incision through the gingival mucosa within the mouth, and opening of the maxillary antrum through its anterolateral wall. The antral mucosa is then carefully removed and an antrostomy fashioned into the nose.

Chronic infection in the ethmoid air cells or in the frontal sinus, is treated first by eliminating disease in the maxillary antrum. Persistent infection in the ethmoid labyrinth may require an ethmoidectomy similar to that described for the management of ethmoid polyps. Persisting *frontal sinusitis* may be surgically treated by an *external frontal operation*.

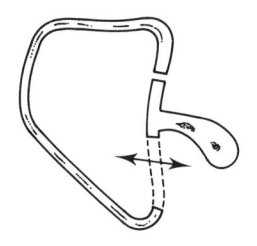

Figure 3.38 Intranasal antrostomy.

Two principles govern the many varieties of this procedure. In one the sinus and its ducts are obliterated completely so there is no remaining air space, while with the other a new wide frontonasal duct is fashioned so that infected material can escape directly into the nose.

Throat diseases

The throat is often blamed, often unjustly, for many local and more distant symptoms.

Locally there are recurring sore throats, persistent cough, loss of voice, throat clearing, snoring and bad breath.

Remotely, throat conditions may be blamed for lethargy and depression and as infective foci for arthritis, endocarditis and nephritis.

Indications for adenotonsillectomy

Adenoidectomy
Adenoidectomy may be required for mechanical reasons of obstruction to the upper airway, or interference with Eustachian-tube function causing secretory otitis media. It may also be indicated for recurrent bacterial infective episodes of the upper respiratory tract in association with bacterial tonsillitis.

Tonsillectomy
This is most often performed because of recurrent bacterial tonsillitis; adenoidectomy is invariably performed at the same time. As mentioned earlier, obstructive sleep apnoea is an additional reason for considering adenotonsillectomy in certain groups of children. Much rarer indications for tonsillectomy and adenoidectomy now include streptococcal allergic disorders such as rheumatic fever, chorea, and type 1 glomerulonephritis.

The indications vary somewhat according to age. Operations should be avoided if at all possible in children below the age of three or four years, since the proportion of total blood volume lost will be greater in a small child than in a larger. Above the age of eight or nine years episodes of bacterial infection decrease in frequency.

Chronic pharyngitis and chronic laryngitis

Chronic inflammation of the upper respiratory tract is always secondary to some irritating factor. This may be persistent mouth breathing with mucosal drying, excessive vocal abuse, smoking, spirit drinking, coughing and recurrent bouts of vomiting. Chronic infection in the sinuses is probably a provoking cause.

Many patients complain of a persisting sore throat without any physical signs of abnormality. A careful history should highlight possible chronic irritating factors. Examination of the pharynx may reveal injection of the faucial pillars, the soft palate and the posterior pharyngeal wall, and there may be hypertrophy of the lymphoid tissue on the posterior pharyngeal wall. The range of variation of appearances however is very great and not clearly related to the symptoms of which a patient complains. Chronic laryngitis can be recognized only by careful indirect laryngoscopy.

Any patient who has been hoarse for more than two or three weeks should be referred for examination of the larynx. In most instances a good mirror view can be obtained (Figure 3.39) and various changes of the vocal cords may be seen. The cords may be red and injected, they may be oedematous with polypoid swelling, there may be fibrous nodules near the anterior end of each cord (*singer's nodes*) usually following vocal abuse. Occasionally whitish keratotic patches of leukoplakia may be seen on the cords. In all instances early referral is necessary to exclude the possibility of malignant disease. If a view cannot be obtained in the outpatient clinic with a laryngeal mirror, the use of a fibreoptic nasolaryngoscope under local anaesthetic may supply a speedy answer. Otherwise the patient may be admitted for examination under general anaesthetic, which is usually conducted through the operating microscope.

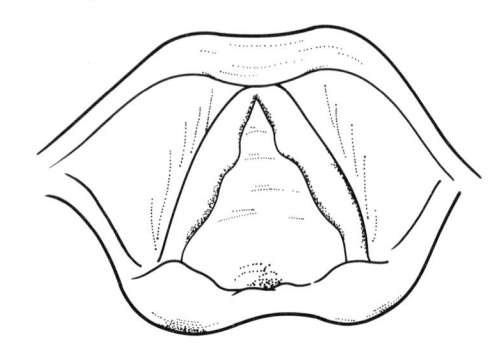

Figure 3.39 View of larynx.

Surgical remedies for chronic laryngitis include the removal of vocal cord redundancies, polyps and fibrous nodules, but in all instances attention to the provoking irritating factors is essential and rehabilitation of the voice with the help of speech therapy may be needed.

Postnasal drip and catarrh

These common complaints are frequently due to misunderstanding about the nature of nasal and paranasal physiology. It is doubtful whether mucus or mucopus ever drips from the postnasal space in the way suspected, and certainly irritation of the larynx by this means is an unrealistic mechanistic explanation.

The term 'catarrh' is used by different patients to describe a multitude of different nasal symptoms, ranging from a runny nose to nasal obstruction. In the normal adult the nose and paranasal sinuses secrete something of the order of 2 litres of mucus in 24 hours and this, after sweeping back into the postnasal space by ciliary action, is swallowed unconsciously.

Almost all the symptoms referred to under these headings stem from minor alterations in the behaviour of the mucociliary blanket. Slight changes in viscosity in the mucus or slight increases in its production may both be responsible for a patient's awareness of the previously unconscious swallowing process. This provokes a complaint.

Some patients become increasingly concerned about the accumulation of this material in the throat and constantly clear their throats in an effort to remove it. Such traumatic irritation provokes further mucus secretion and exacerbates the condition. A clear understanding by the doctor, and careful explanation to the patient will resolve many of the problems. Medical treatment and surgical remedies are almost always inappropriate.

Persisting unproductive cough

The patient is usually a child who has suffered some sort of upper respiratory tract viral infection and for several months afterwards has had a barking, dry cough. This causes considerable alarm even though no chest abnormalities can be demonstrated. A similar pattern is occasionally seen in adults, and again usually follows an upper respiratory tract viral infection.

Careful examination of the upper respiratory tract rarely reveals any abnormality, and x-rays of the sinuses to exclude sinus disease are invariably normal.

It seems probable that the upper respiratory tract mucosa may be damaged by certain viral infections and take many months to recover. In these circumstances the cough reflex may be triggered by stimuli that were previously below its threshold. Recovery can take many months.

This is not a surgical problem, but simple measures such as the use of cough suppressants, antihistamine tablets, and steroid nasal and throat sprays may all help to suppress the symptom.

Some persistent coughs in young children are believed to be a form of 'asthma' and may be relieved by antispasmodics such as salbutamol, but some coughs are thought to be psychogenic.

Early malignant disease

The early symptoms of malignant disease of ear, nose and throat present problems and challenges, since they may appear identical to common benign conditions.

Paranasal sinuses

Malignant tumours in this site are usually squamous cell carcinomas occurring in middle to old age. They should be suspected in patients who develop chronic sinusitis, without obvious cause, for the first time in later life.

As the tumour grows it extends beyond the bony walls of the ethmoid and the maxillary sinuses and causes swelling of the face, displacement of the eye with proptosis and diplopia, nasal obstruction with blood-stained discharge, and swelling of the palate with loosening of the teeth.

Examination of the nose may reveal friable vascular material from which biopsy specimens can be taken.

Investigation requires radiography with tomograms, or high-resolution CT scanning to show erosion of bone. These tumours rarely spread to regional lymph nodes.

Treatment includes surgical excision of parts of the maxilla and sinuses, combined with radiotherapy, and sometimes cytotoxic drugs. The 5-year survival depends on the site and extent of the tumour, but 30 per cent would be a rough overall figure.

Postnasal carcinoma

This is a rare form of malignant disease in developed countries. Most tumours of the postnasal space are squamous cell carcinomas. Spread of disease within the postnasal space may cause nasal obstruction and bleeding. Metastatic spread to lymph nodes may lead to presentation with a swelling in the neck (Figure 3.40). Invasion of the tissue around the Eustachian orifice may cause Eustachian tube obstruction with an effusion in the middle ear on that side and a conductive hearing loss. This is an important form of presentation, and the diagnosis must be

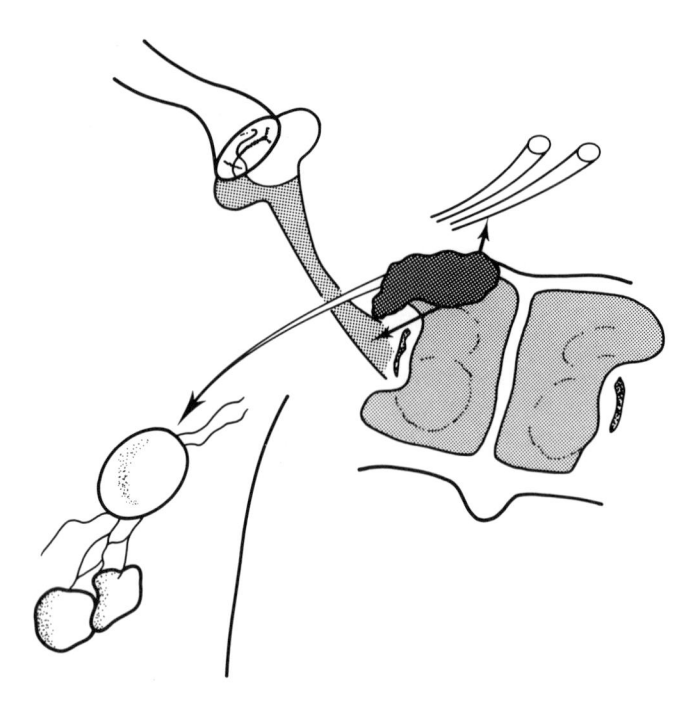

Figure 3.40 Spread of postnasal carcinoma.

considered a possibility in any adult presenting with secretory otitis media. Invasion of the muscles of the soft palate may cause impairment of speech and nasal regurgitation. Upward extension of the tumour in the region of the apex of the petrous temporal bone may affect the trigeminal nerve with pain in the face, and nerves to the external ocular muscles with diplopia and strabismus. More rarely, backward extension on the base of the skull can involve lower cranial nerves (IXth, Xth, and XIth).

Suspicion of the possibility of postnasal carcinoma demands urgent referral to an ENT Department where the postnasal space can be examined with a postnasal mirror. Unsatisfactory viewing of that region with a mirror often requires examination under a general anaesthetic, and sometimes biopsy through an apparently intact and normal mucosa.

Treatment is by external irradiation, sometimes combined with chemotherapy. The only role for surgery would be an excision of neck lymph nodes if a primary has been cured. Overall 5-year survival rate is about 25 per cent.

Malignant disease of the larynx

These tumours, far commoner in men than in women, are usually squamous cell carcinomas. They are classified according to their site of origin into glottic from vocal cords, supraglottic from the region above the cords, and subglottic from below the cords (Figure 3.41).

Glottic carcinomas present early with hoarseness and, because lymphatic spread is late, they have the best prognosis.

Supraglottic carcinomas may extend to a considerable size before causing hoarseness or affecting the airway, while subglottic tumours may present for the first time with difficulty in

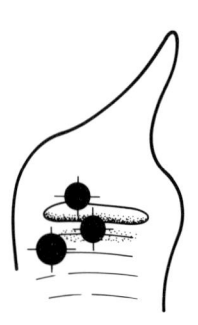

Figure 3.41 Sites of carcinoma of larynx.

breathing from obstruction of the subglottic lumen. The essential investigation for any of these tumours is urgent referral for examination of the larynx.

Treatment of laryngeal tumours is often first by external irradiation, with or without chemotherapy. Some tumours, especially after failure of cure by irradiation, need laryngectomy or partial laryngectomy, and radical neck dissection may be advisable. Five-year survival rates range from over 95 per cent for early glottic tumours to 30 per cent for some subglottic lesions.

Malignant tumours of the laryngopharynx

These may be classified according to the site of origin into pyriform fossa, postcricoid (Figure 3.42), and posterior and lateral pharyngeal walls – the latter are by far the rarest.

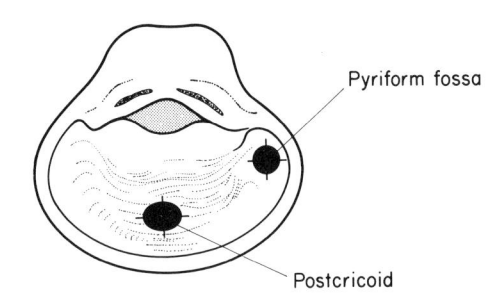

Figure 3.42 Malignant tumours of the laryngopharynx.

Postcricoid carcinoma

Postcricoid carcinoma is the only tumour more prevalent in women. It occurs in middle-aged women suffering from the Paterson–Kelly (Plummer–Vinson) syndrome, with iron deficiency anaemia, koilonychia, glossitis and angular stomatitis. The development of a malignant tumour at the postcricoid site is preceded for some years by a fibrous web of scar tissue under the atrophic postcricoid mucosa. The symptoms of this tumour are difficulty in swallowing, which has often been preceded by the complaint of many years of 'small swallow'. Investigation requires endoscopy after barium swallow, and biopsy of any tumour mass.

Tumours of the pyriform fossa

These are commoner in men than in women, and may present with enlargement of a lymph node in the neck. They do not cause dysphagia until very large, since there is much more room in the region of the two pyriform fossae for the passage of a food bolus. A presenting symptom is pain referred to the ear. Invasion of the muscles of the larynx medial to the pyriform fossa causes hoarseness. As with all the other tumours in the larynx, and at these sites of the laryngopharynx, investigation demands referral for examination with a laryngeal mirror, possible endoscopy, and biopsy.

The prognosis of postcricoid tumours is so poor (less than 5 per cent 5-year survival rate) that any treatment should be considered palliative. Options include external irradiation with chemotherapy, or surgical excision – pharyngolaryngectomy – with reconstruction of the gullet. Pyriform fossa tumours have only a slightly better prognosis, and similar treatment options are available.

General concluding comments

It is accepted that the general practitioner has limited time and equipment to deal in any detail with ENT diseases. However, as an expert general clinician, the general practitioner is in an important position to make decisions on what to treat, and what to refer to the consultant.

In this chapter some selected diseases have been described to illustrate these points.

4 Lumps in the Neck

Hedley E. Berry and John Fry

Lumps in the neck are common. They may range from 'normal abnormalities' such as lymph nodes that are palpable in all children between three and eight years of age, through a number of conditions, to highly malignant neoplastic tumours.

In this chapter we do not attempt to give a comprehensive account of all possible lumps in the neck, but to highlight practical points to enable a clinical diagnosis to be made.

General principles

The most likely swellings in the neck are lymph nodes (Figure 4.1) and the most likely causes of lymphadenopathy are infections and metastatic spread of cancer.

```
              Neck swellings
             /      |      \
            /       |       \
      Lymph nodes  Goitres  Others
         85%        8%       7%
```

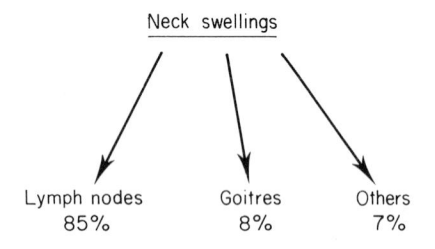

Figure 4.1 Causes of neck swellings.

Lymph nodes are recognized by their physical signs more easily when multiple than when solitary. It is the solitary lymph node that presents the greatest diagnostic challenges.

Goitres are dealt with in Chapter 5.
Solitary nodules in the thyroid are distinguished from other lumps in the neck by the fact that they move on swallowing.
Swellings which arise in the *skin* are not considered, but routine examination of every lump must elicit whether the skin is involved. Sebaceous cysts can occur anywhere and are part of the skin structure. The diagnosis of a lipoma may be difficult when it is subfascial, and often depends on its excision and histological examination.

Systemic symptoms such as fever, weight loss, or sweats must be noted, since they may point to a possible generalized condition such as glandular fever, lymphoma, thyrotoxicosis, tuberculosis or other infections.

Specific symptoms such as hoarseness, cough, or shortness of breath may suggest the site of a primary tumour.

Examination must extend beyond the neck, and include lymphatic fields elsewhere and the abdomen for enlargement of the liver and spleen, if lymphoproliferative disease is suspected. An abdominal mass may indicate the site of a primary tumour.

The patient's background, particularly if a recent immigrant or overseas traveller, may make diagnosis of tuberculosis or tropical disease possible.

Anatomical location of an enlarged lymph node wil be a guide to its underlying cause, and if infective or neoplastic. Hence, a knowledge of areas drained by lymph nodes is important. Anatomical knowledge is also essential in identifying such specific conditions as branchial and thyroglossal cysts which occupy characteristic positions.

Age at presentation is helpful. Branchial and thyroglossal cysts are congenital and may be noted in infancy, but they may sometimes not appear until advanced age.

Infections are most common in childhood from foci in the throat and ears.

Teenagers are prone to glandular fever (infectious mononucleosis). Lymphomata and lymphoproliferative disease can occur at any age and are not uncommon in young and middle-aged adults.

Neoplastic diseases are to be expected more in the elderly, but can be found at any age.

Cervical lymphadenopathy (Figure 4.2)

Always:

1. Look for other nodes at distant sites
2. Look for possible primary source of infection or neoplasia
3. Look for liver and spleen enlargement.

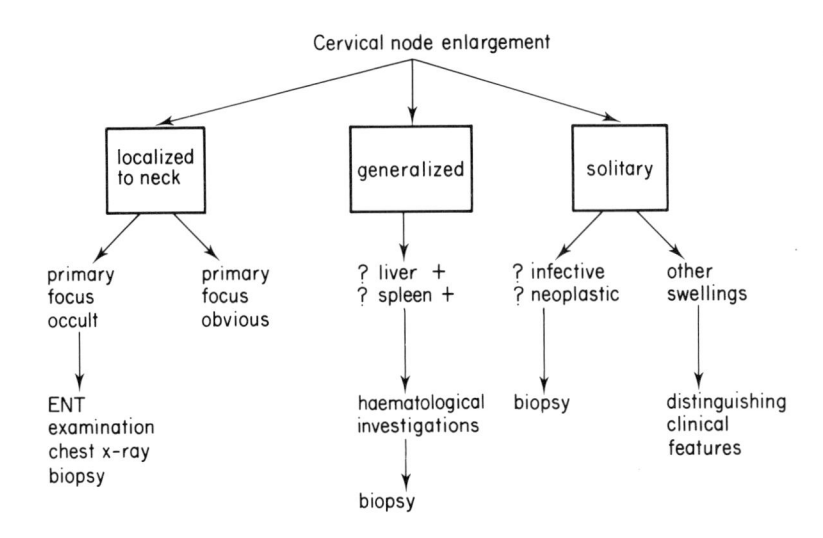

Figure 4.2 Cervical lymphadenopathy.

Infective lymph nodes

Infective lymph nodes are either acute and painful or chronic painful/painless.

Acute and painful

Consider:
 Staphlyococcal infection
 Streptococcal infection
 Glandular fever
 'Reactive' lymph nodes.

The fact that the node(s) are acute and painful may be obvious, the exact diagnosis may not be so.

There may be primary foci in the throat, ears or skin to suggest common pathogenic organisms, but no such focus may be apparent. Often it is necessary to manage such patients without confirmation of the causal organisms, and treat with antibiotics.

Painful neck glands in the young should always raise the possibility of glandular fever, and

40 Lumps in the neck

appropriate blood tests carried out.

'Reactive' lymph nodes is a diagnosis of exclusion, when no reason can be found and swelling persists after treatment and observation. The diagnosis has to be made as a result of biopsy.

Chronic and painless/painful

Tuberculosis of cervical lymph nodes is not rare. Although more common in immigrants from Asian or African countries, it can occur in indigents at any age. In the early stages a discrete, firm, localized lymphadenopathy is the rule, and at this stage distinction from metastatic carcinoma usually requires biopsy. Later the nodes coalesce, caseation and cold-abscess formation occurs. At a late stage distinction from a branchial cyst (vide infra) may be difficult. Aspiration of tuberculous pus will enable a diagnosis to be made, and the sensitivity of the organism to various antibiotics can be determined.

Metastatic lymph nodes

Anatomical site of enlargement will provide clues as to cause (Figure 4.3).

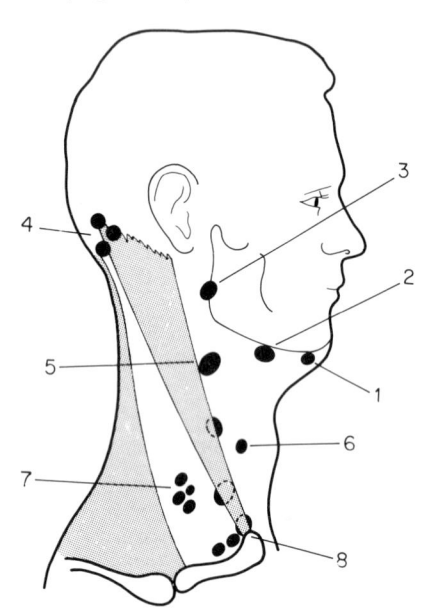

Figure 4.3 Metastatic lymph nodes.

Left supraclavicular node enlargement (8) (Troisier's sign) occurs in patients with carcinoma of the stomach.
    Occipital nodes (4) – look at scalp.
    Upper deep cervical (5) – check tonsils.
    Submental (1) – check tongue, teeth and mouth.
    Submandibular (2) – check floor of mouth.
    Preparotid (3) – check parotid gland and ear.
    Check thyroid (6).
    Tuberculous nodes can occur anywhere, but particularly in posterior triangle (7) and upper deep cervical (5).

Check sites of possible occult, symptomless primary tumours (Figure 4.4):

    Mouth
    Pharynx
    Sinuses
    Larynx
    Scalp
    Oesophagus
    Stomach
    Breast
    Thyroid
    Lung

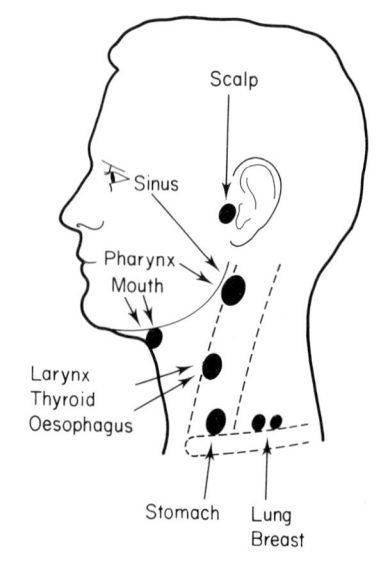

Figure 4.4 Occult, symptomless primary tumours.

Biopsy is often required to establish the diagnosis firmly. Open biopsy as opposed to needle biopsy is usually preferred, and frozen section examination may be valuable if block dissection is contemplated. Very often the pathologist will be unable to indicate the site of the primary tumour.

Lymphoproliferative disease

Under this heading are included all malignant conditions arising in lymph nodes. They fall into two main groups: the leukaemias, and the lymphomas which are further subdivided into Hodgkin's lymphomas and nonHodgkin's lymphomas (Figure 4.5).

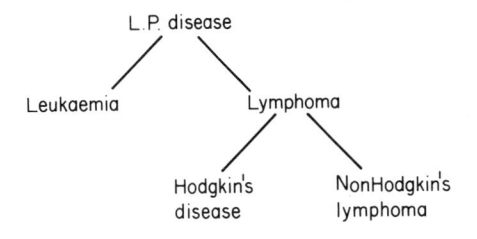

Figure 4.5 Lymphoproliferative disease.

The improving prognosis for patients suffering from lymphoma reflects not only improving treatment with radiotherapy and especially chemotherapy, but also the efforts made in recent years to stage and classify the disease more accurately.

The commonest form of lymphoma is Hodgkin's disease (Figure 4.6) which most often afflicts young males. It usually presents with discrete, rubbery, painless nodes especially in the neck but it may be a generalized disease with systemic symptoms at the time it presents.

The surgeon's role mainly concerns the diagnosis and staging of the lymphomas (Figure 4.7). Node biopsy should, whenever possible, include a whole lymph node taken from the largest group. This enables the pathologist to give an accurate histological classification, which is an important guide to treatment and prognosis. Four main types are described: lymphocyte predominant, nodular sclerotic, mixed cellular, and lymphocyte depleted. About 40 per cent of patients with lymphocyte predominant disease can be expected to survive fifteen years, compared to less than 5 per cent of those with lymphocyte depleted disease.

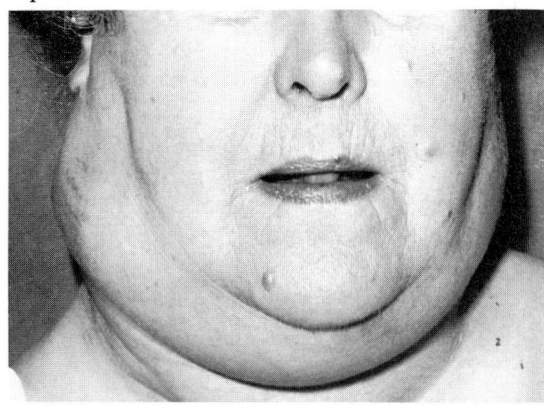

Figure 4.6 Hodgkin's nodes in the neck.

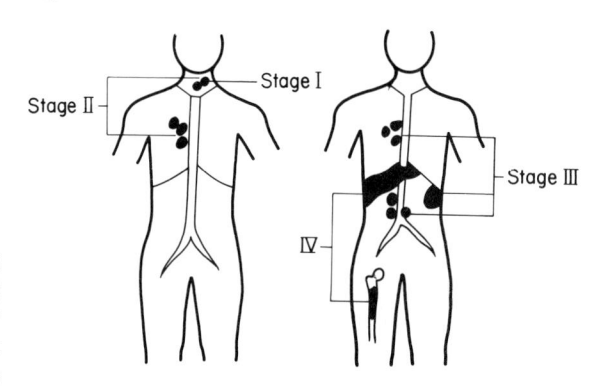

Figure 4.7
Clinical staging of Hodgkin's disease.
Stage I: Single node region involved;
Stage II: Two node regions on same side of diaphragm involved;
Stage III: Nodes involved on both sides of diaphragm ± spleen;
Stage IV: Diffuse involvement of extranodal sites (bone, liver, etc.).

In addition to node biopsy, examination of the peripheral blood, chest x-ray, skeletal survey, and bone-marrow biopsy are performed as routine. Lymphangiography may give an indication of involvement of abdominal and thoracic lymph nodes.

The surgeon may also be called upon to undertake a laparotomy to obtain biopsy material from abdominal nodes and to remove the spleen. The indications for laparotomy, however, are decreasing with the improved techniques of computerized tomography.

Swellings in the neck from which an isolated enlarged lymph node must be distinguished

Midline swellings (Figure 4.8)

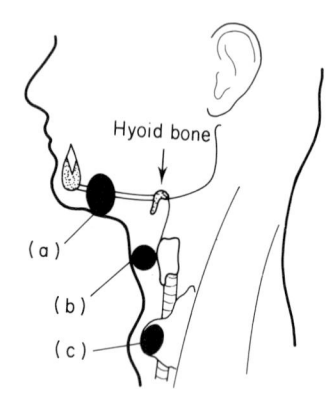

Figure 4.8 Relationship of swellings to the hyoid bone.

When examining midline swellings, determine first the relationship to the hyoid bone and whether there is any attachment to the bone. Suprahyoid swellings may be palpable sublingually in the mouth (a). A thyroglossal cyst (b) will move upwards on protruding the tongue; a thyroid swelling (c) will move on swallowing.

Thyroid swellings
An adenoma or cyst arising in the isthmus of the thyroid gland presents as a midline swelling which, unlike other swellings, moves on swallowing. These swellings can occur at any age and usually present no difficulty in diagnosis, except that of distinguishing an enlarged pretracheal 'delphic' lymph node which is attached to the isthmus.

Thyroglossal cysts (Figure 4.9)
Thyroglossal cysts may arise in any part of the thyroglossal tract, which extends from the isthmus of the thyroid gland to the tongue. They are most commonly seen just below the level of the hyoid bone, to which attachment by the tract may be demonstrated. When situated at the level of the thyroid cartilage (b) the cyst is usually deviated to one side, most often to the left. The lower, pretracheal variety (a) may be difficult to distinguish from swellings in the thyroid isthmus and a suprahyoid cyst (c) may be clinically indistinguishable from a sublingual dermoid cyst.

Thyroglossal cysts (Figure 4.10) commonly present at the age of fifteen to twenty years but they can occur at any age. Upward movement on protrusion of the tongue is a diagnostic feature.

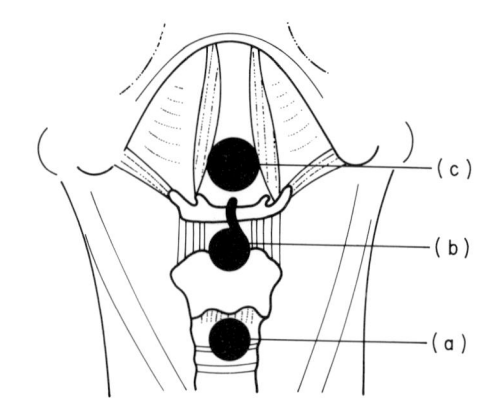

Figure 4.9 Locations of thyroglossal cysts.

The wall contains lymphatic tissue which may transmit infection, causing the cyst to present as an acute abscess. Infection usually responds to antibiotics when treated early but if surgical drainage is required a thyroglossal fistula can result.

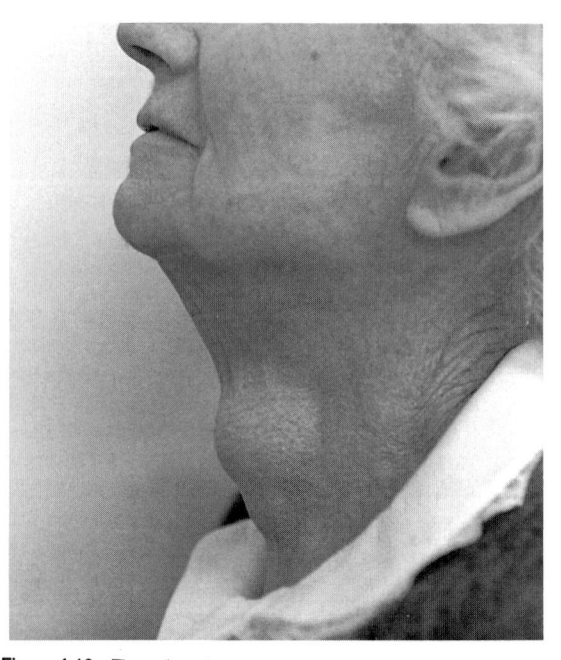

Figure 4.10 Thyroglossal cyst.

Dermoid cysts

Dermoid cysts (Figure 4.11) usually occur in teenagers and young adults; although congenital they do not often appear in infancy.

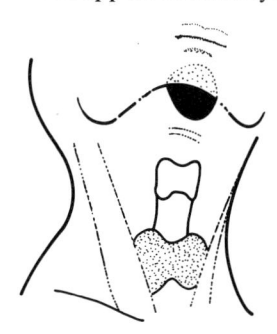

Figure 4.11 Dermoid cyst.

A soft, fluctuant, midline swelling enlarges gradually beneath the chin. It seldom becomes inflamed.

These cysts arise above or below the mylohyoid muscle. When above (sublingual dermoid cyst) they can attain an extraordinary size before they present as a swelling displacing the tongue upwards. When large they may extend through the floor of the mouth to cause swelling beneath the chin, perhaps only apparent when the mouth is closed.

Cysts below the mylohyoid produce an appearance often complained of as a double chin. The swelling, anterior to the hyoid bone, needs to be distinguished from a suprahyoid thyroglossal cyst or an ectopic thyroid gland.

Dermoid cysts enlarge as time goes on and should be referred for excision.

Anterior triangle

Branchial cyst

A branchial cyst (Figure 4.12) is thought to be a remnant of the developmental system of the branchial clefts and arches in the early embryo. This does not explain, however, why it does not normally present until adult life.

These cysts are usually sited in the upper part of the anterior triangle, at the junction of the upper third and lower two-thirds of the anterior border of the sternomastoid. They may appear to overlie the sternomastoid, but getting the patient to contract the muscle will establish that the posterior part of the cyst is deep. When large they may extend high into the neck and be difficult to distinguish from a parotid-gland swelling. Large cysts are usually soft and fluctuant, but smaller ones may appear solid, and the proximity to the carotid artery raises the possibility of a carotid body tumour, especially if pulsation is transmitted.

When firm the differential diagnosis includes lymphadenopathy, and when soft and fluctuant a branchial cyst may mimic a 'cold' abscess of caseating tuberculous nodes. Aspiration distinguishes the two; a tuberculous abscess contains caseous material and a cyst yellow fluid containing cholesterol.

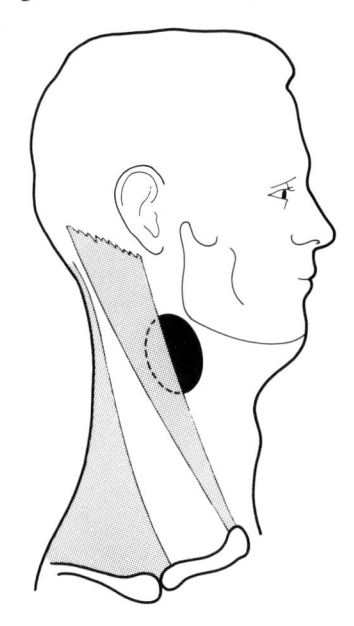

Figure 4.12 Branchial cyst.

Because branchial cysts contain lymphatic tissue in communication with the tonsillar region, they sometimes present as an acute abscess following a sore throat. If they can be distinguished from a suppurative adenitis, they should be treated with antibiotics because incision and drainage make subsequent removal of the cyst more difficult.

Carotid body tumour (potato tumour, chemodectoma)

Carotid body tumours (Figure 4.13) usually present in middle-age (40–60 years), the patient most often having a visible swelling in the neck which may have been increasing in size for years. The symptomless lump, 3–5 cm in diameter, is always situated beneath the edge of the sternomastoid at the level of the hyoid bone. It is hard and elastic in consistency, and classically moves laterally but not vertically. Pulsation of the overlying external carotid artery may be obvious, but often less so than the pulsation transmitted, for example, by an overlying lymphadenopathy.

The possibility of a carotid body tumour should always be borne in mind when lumps closely related to the carotid artery are found, and the surgeon should avoid the dangerous procedure of biopsy at this site. Angiography and ultrasound examination will facilitate diagnosis.

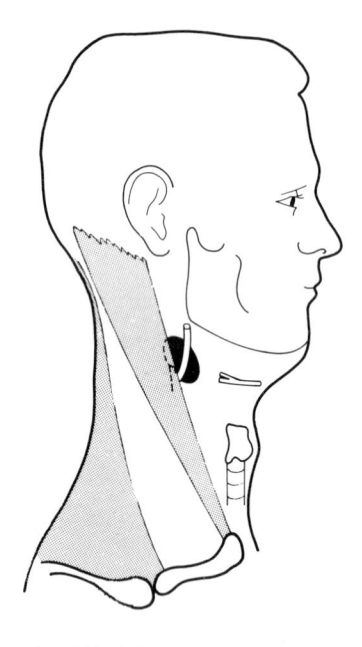

Figure 4.13 Carotid body tumour.

Carotid body tumours should always be excised, except perhaps in the very elderly. Early tumours may be removed by separating them from the carotid vessels, but larger tumours usually involve arterial grafting.

Carotid aneurysm
Carotid artery aneurysms are very rare. The majority are due to atherosclerosis and are therefore most often seen in the elderly. They usually occur at the bifurcation of the common carotid artery, where they present as a painful, pulsating lump, which has to be distinguished from a carotid body tumour or enlarged lymph nodes. A systolic bruit is usually audible over the aneurysm. Untreated, carotid aneurysms are hazardous lesions because the incidence of rupture and cerebral embolism is high. The diagnosis is made by angiography.

Tortuous carotid artery
Tortuosity and buckling of the carotid arteries is fairly commonly seen, usually on the right side of the neck in elderly female hypertensive patients. It may simulate a carotid aneurysm and arteriography may be required to distinguish the two. Tortuosity is of little prognostic significance and requires no treatment.

Nodules in the lateral thyroid
These may present as lumps in the anterior triangle of the neck (Figure 4.14) and are fully described in Chapter 5. Movement on swallowing distinguishes them from other lumps.

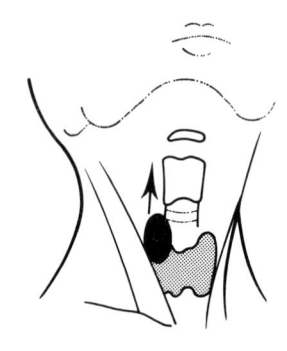

Figure 4.14 Nodules in the lateral thyroid.

Posterior triangle

Cystic hygroma and lymphatic cysts
The majority of cystic hygromas appear in the first year of life when they may grow rapidly to such a size as to cause severe pressure symptoms in the neck.

Solitary lymphatic cysts occasionally present in adult life as a soft fluctuant, superficial swelling above the clavicle (Figure 4.15). They occur

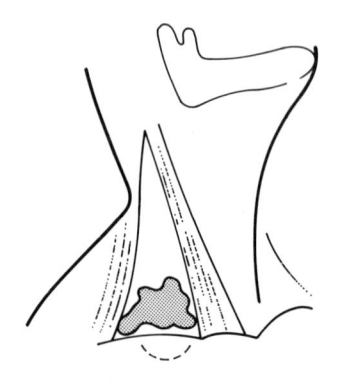

Figure 4.15 Cystic hygroma.

superficial to the muscles and close to the skin, with the result that they brilliantly transilluminate. Excision is satisfactory.

Pancoast's tumour
These are usually poorly differentiated squamous carcinomas arising in the apex of the lung. A supraclavicular mass situated in the posterior triangle may be palpable. Involvement of the brachial plexus may produce intractable pain, and sympathetic-chain invasion results in a Horner's syndrome.

Cervical rib
A cervical rib (Figure 4.16) may present as a hard, fixed swelling above the clavicle in the posterior triangle of the neck. There may be a visible fullness of the neck and on palpation the rib may be mistaken for a mass of malignant lymph nodes. The subclavian artery may be pushed forwards and be palpable as a pulsatile swelling in the posterior triangle. Present in only 1 per cent of the population, only 10 per cent of cervical ribs cause symptoms. When they do, pressure on the brachial plexus causes neurological symptoms, or vascular complications may occur because the subclavian artery is embarrassed. Symptoms can be relieved in the majority of patients by attention to posture and the avoidance of carrying heavy weights.

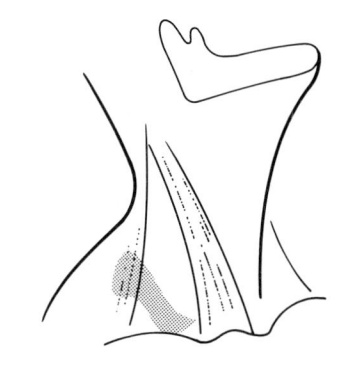

Figure 4.16 Cervical rib.

Subclavian artery aneurysm
Anerurysms of the subclavian artery are most often associated with congenital lesions, such as a cervical rib producing compression of the artery leading to post-stenotic dilatation and aneurysm formation. They may present as a pulsating supraclavicular mass.

Submandibular swellings

Examination of the oral cavity is essential in any patient who presents with a swelling in the submandibular triangle. Enlargement of the submandibular salivary gland is the commonest cause of such a swelling and this must be distinguished from a lymphadenopathy secondary to infection or neoplasm in the mouth. Caries and dental-root infections may underlie the node enlargement and the teeth should be checked in the absence of other obvious lesions.

Submandibular salivary gland

The commonest cause of enlargement is obstruction of Wharton's duct. This may occur secondary to a stricture of the duct, a tumour in the mouth or an ill-fitting denture leading to ulceration of the papilla; but by far the commonest cause is a submandibular calculus.

Calculi occur most commonly in young adults and the diagnosis is usually easy because the complaint is of recurrent painful swelling with meals. The visible swelling in the neck has often subsided by the time the patient presents but an enlarged gland may still be palpable bidigitally. A calculus is often palpable with the finger just proximal to the duct papilla. Occasionally, difficulties in diagnosis arise because a calculus is not palpable and the gland presents as a persistent swelling due to subacute infection.

Even if a calculus is easily palpable in the floor of the mouth, a plain radiograph should be taken because this may demonstrate additional calculi in the proximal duct or in the gland itself (Figure 4.17).

A sialogram (Figure 4.18) may be taken to demonstrate the duct system and to show any obstructions.

Stones in the anterior part of the duct can be removed by incision of the duct in the floor of the mouth. When the gland itself contains stones or is damaged by recurrent infection, then excision of the whole gland is required.

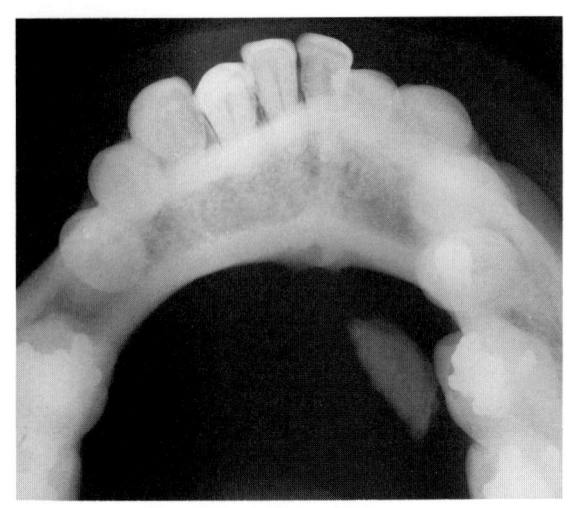

Figure 4.17 Plain radiograph showing calculi.

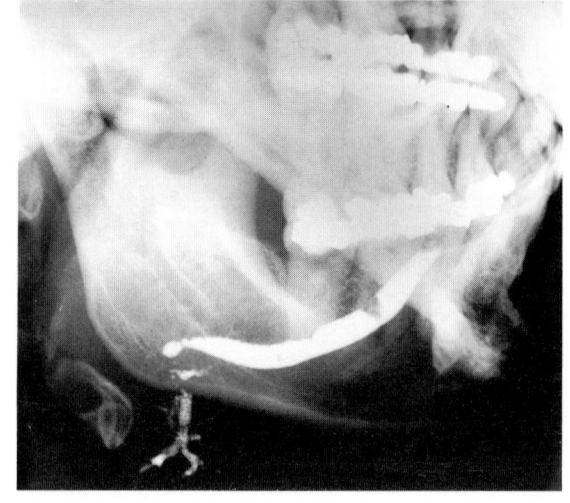

Figure 4.18 Sialogram.

Salivary gland tumours

A full account of salivary gland tumours is beyond the scope of this chapter. The majority arise in the parotid gland, but it should be remembered that approximately 15 per cent arise in the submandibular salivary gland, of which the majority are pleomorphic adenomas ('mixed' salivary tumours). These slow-growing tumours may have been present for years, but the long history should not reassure the doctor because rapid growth and malignant change can occur. Persistent enlargement of the submandibular gland, even when symptomless, must be referred for surgical excision. Excision of the gland must be complete, and biopsies are never taken because of the risk of shedding cells.

5 Thyroid Disorders

Hedley E. Berry and John Fry

Introduction

Thyroid disease is not infrequent in the community.

A general practitioner with 2500 patients can expect one new case of thyroid disease each year, and at any time have for care and follow-up 10–15 persons with a past or present thyroid disorder.

A district general hospital will receive 50–100 new cases of thyroid disease annually, with larger numbers attending for supervision (if that is its policy).

Thyroid disorders can occur at any *age* but most frequently present in early adulthood and middle-age.

Types of thyroid disease in a general practice are likely to be as shown in Table 5.1.

Table 5.1 Incidence of thyroid disease.

	per 2500 over 20 years
euthyroid goitre	5
hyperthyroid	8
hypothyroid	7
cancer	1

Early symptoms and signs of disordered thyroid function

Early symptoms and signs often go unrecognized, possibly because they present in a manner which does not bring the diagnosis of thyroid disorder to mind. Presenting features may relate to any clinical specialty.

Hyperthyroidism

In addition to classical symptoms of weight loss, sweating, and heat intolerance, there may be:

psychiatric symptoms
  anxiety; irritability; depression

cardiological symptoms
  rapid pulse
  palpitations; auricular fibrillation (especially in the elderly, and often with no palpable thyroid swelling)
  heart failure, particularly in the elderly

neurological symptoms
  tremor
  brisk reflexes

rheumatological symptoms
  weakness
  aches and pains in limbs, in muscles and joints

gastroenterological symptoms
  increased appetite
  diarrhoea

gynaecological symptoms
  menses may be more frequent and heavier, but amenorrhoea may occur

dermatological symptoms
  hands are hot and moist
  nail changes

ophthalmological symptoms
  exophthalmos, which may become malignant.

Hypothyroidism

This is more difficult to diagnose than hyperthyroidism; there may be long delays with well known patients. Often a partner or locum may suspect or diagnose the condition.

psychiatric symptoms
  tiredness; no 'go'
  poor memory
  depression; dullness; slowness
  irritability
  changes in appearance (becoming coarse and unattractive)
  frank psychosis (rare)

cardiological symptoms
  slow pulse
  angina on effort
  breathlessness

neurological symptoms
  paraesthesia in hands (carpal tunnel syndrome)
  slow reflexes

rheumatological symptoms
  weakness of muscles
  aching joints

laryngeal symptoms
  voice changes

gastrointestinal symptoms
  constipation

gynaecological symptoms
  amenorrhoea
  heavy menses
  infertility

skin symptoms
  coarseness; dry and thickened

scalp symptoms
  thinning hair and dry scalp

symptoms in infancy
  neonatal jaundice
  retarded progress
  'cretinism'; mental dullness.

In surgery, **hyperthyroidism** is the chief concern of the clinician.

The investigation of disturbed thyroid function

The days are past when the diagnosis of disturbed thyroid function depended on clinical history and examination. The use of radioactive isotopes and radioimmunoassay allows accurate estimation of thyroid function. Nevertheless, there are pitfalls in the interpretation of thyroid function studies, and the investigation of many patients suspected of having thyroid disorders will yield equivocal results which may be influenced by extrathyroidal factors that must be recognized. Correct interpretation of thyroid function tests depends upon understanding current knowledge of the thyroid physiology on which the tests are based (Figure 5.1).

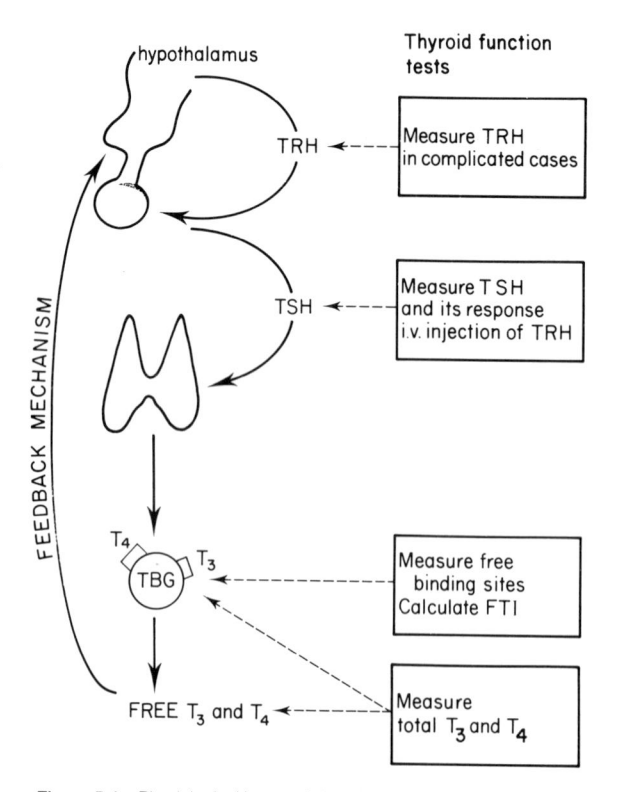

Figure 5.1 Physiological bases of thyroid function tests.

Iodine

This is ingested chiefly in fish and dairy products, and is absorbed from the stomach and small intestine as iodide (I^-). Iodide is concentrated chiefly in the thyroid gland, where it is bound to

Disordered thyroid function

tyrosine, which is in turn coupled to form thyroxine (T_4) and triiodothyronine (T_3) (Figure 5.2).

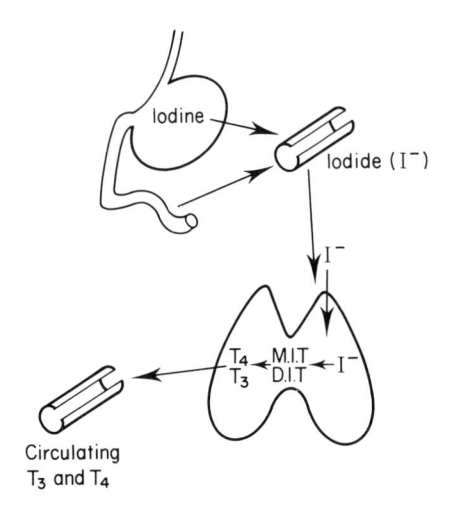

Figure 5.2 Thyroid physiology.

Thyroid function tests

The measurement of protein-bound iodine (PBI) is no longer employed because it is subject to inaccuracies, when for example serum protein levels are low, or when the patient has received iodine in radiological studies during preceding months. Radioactive iodine uptake tests have also been largely superseded in the diagnosis of thyroid disorders.

The release of T_3 and T_4 is controlled by a feedback mechanism (Figure 5.3). Low circulating levels of T_3 and T_4 stimulate the release of thyrotrophin-releasing hormone (TRH) by the hypothalamus and this in turn brings about the release of thyrotrophin-stimulating hormone (TSH) by the pituitary. Circulating levels of TSH can now be assayed. Levels are suppressed in thyrotoxicosis and elevated in myxoedema.

Serum TSH

The main value of estimating serum TSH is to distinguish between myxoedema due to primary thyroid failure and that due to pituitary failure. In the former the TSH level is elevated, but in pituitary failure it is depressed. The estimation of TSH may also be of value in the *early* diagnosis of disordered thyroid function, when serum T_3 and T_4 levels may be equivocal. After thyroid surgery the early diagnosis of myxoedema may be recognized by an elevation in the TSH.

TRH test

This may be of value in ruling out thyrotoxicosis when clinical assessment is difficult and the routine tests give equivocal results. An intravenous injection of TRH normally results in the release of TSH from the pituitary. No response is expected in thyrotoxicosis and a positive response rules it out.

Only a small proportion of T_3 and T_4 is free and biologically active in the serum. The majority is bound to the protein carrier thyroid binding globulin (TBG) (Figure 5.4).

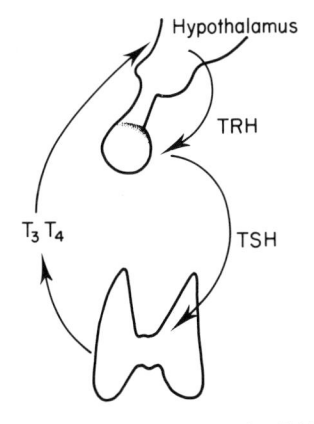

Figure 5.3 Triiodothyronine (T_3) and thyroxine (T_4) feedback mechanism.

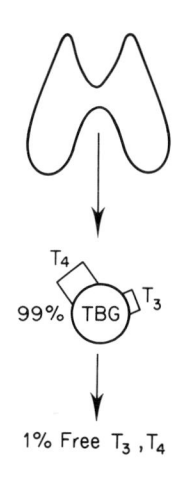

Figure 5.4 Distribution of T_3 and T_4.

Serum T_4

Ideally, the active free T_4 in the serum should be measured, but this estimation is not freely available. A patient who is euthyroid will have normal levels of circulating *free* T_4, but the *total* T_4 which is usually measured may be abnormally high or low because of an excess or deficiency of circulating TBG.

Serum T_3

Serum T_3 estimations can now be done, and are important in those rare cases when the thyroid gland preferentially secretes T_3. If the clinical diagnosis is convincing and the T_4 level is normal, a T_3 estimation should be requested.

More than 99 per cent of circulating T_4 is protein bound. When levels of TBG are high, elevated T_4 levels will be obtained and a spurious diagnosis of 'thyrotoxicosis' may be made in a patient who has normal circulating levels of free T_4. This is commonly the cause of equivocal results in patients taking an oestrogen-containing contraceptive pill (Figure 5.5). Further thyroid function tests are necessary to clarify the diagnosis.

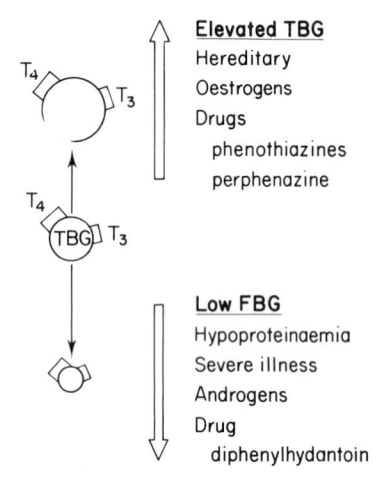

Figure 5.5 Factors affecting TBG.

Free thyroxine index (FTI)

Free thyroxine index estimations make it possible to correct for variations in TBG and are important in patients taking drugs which influence TBG, especially oestrogen-containing oral contraceptives. In these cases a marginally elevated serum T_4 must be supported by a raised FTI before a confident diagnosis of thyrotoxicosis can be made. The concentration of unoccupied binding sites on TBG is estimated by adding radioactive T_4 to the patient's serum.

The free thyroxine index is calculated as

$$\text{FTI} = \frac{\text{serum } T_4 \times 100}{T_3 \text{ resin uptake } \%}$$

The FTI for T_3 can also be estimated by the use of radioactive T_3.

A high T_3 value is almost always found in hyperthyroidism, and a low value in myxoedema. T_4 values near the upper end of the normal range must be supported by an elevated FTI before treatment for thyrotoxicosis is commenced. Many normal individuals have an undetectably low TSH level. Most laboratories routinely estimate TSH levels in patients with T_4 levels below 60 nmol/litre. In hypothroidism it is usually greater than 20 m units/litre, and in severe cases may exceed 300 m units/litre.

See Table 5.2 for normal values.

Table 5.2 Thyroid profile — normal values

T_4	55–150	nmol/litre
T_3	1.3–3.5	nmol/litre
FT4I	55–155	nmol/litre
FT3I	1.4–3.7	nmol/litre
TSH	range 4–10	m units/litre

The thyroid nodule

The majority of patients with thyroid disorders present with a *lump in the neck*. Initial clinical evaluation of these patients will enable them to be divided broadly into two groups.

A careful history will distinguish those patients who have symptoms referable to the goitre. This group will more often prove to have *diffuse thyroid disease*: hyperthyroidism, multinodular goitre, thyroiditis, or occasionally extensive carcinoma (Figure 5.6).

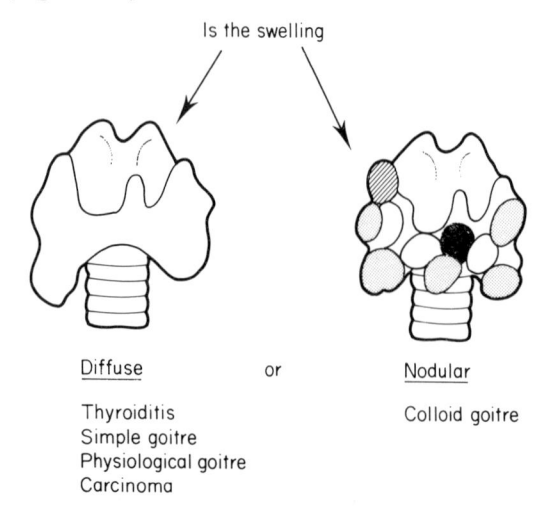

Figure 5.6 Clinical examination of an enlarged thyroid gland.

The second group are asymptomatic and often prove to have a well circumscribed lesion in the thyroid gland. This may be a cyst, a benign adenoma or a carcinoma. It is in this group that the burden of proof (to rule out malignancy) lies with the clinician.

Assessment of the patient with an enlarged thyroid gland must initially attempt to answer the following questions:

Is the patient

EUTHYROID?

THYROTOXIC?

HYPOTHYROID?

The clinician must be alert to the early symptoms and signs of disordered thyroid function. Investigation must always include estimation of the serum thyroxine (T_4), and T_3 when indicated.

In the *euthyroid patient* the differential diagnosis has to be made between three conditions: Hashimoto's disease, malignancy, and goitre.

Hashimoto's disease or autoimmune thyroiditis

This usually presents with a firm, diffuse enlargement of the whole gland. However, the enlargement may be predominantly in one lobe of the gland and the distinction from a carcinoma can be difficult on clinical grounds alone. The diagnosis rests on finding a high level of circulating thyroid antibodies in the serum. In the early stages it may be associated with mild thyrotoxicosis and in the late stages myxoedema is frequent.

Malignancy (anaplastic carcinoma)

This may occasionally present as a diffuse enlargement of the whole gland and should be suspected if there is a rapid increase in size of the gland, if the gland is painful, or if there is hoarseness due to involvement of the recurrent laryngeal nerve.

Physiological goitre

A soft difffuse enlargement of the whole gland occurs in girls at puberty, in pregnancy and at the menopause. Spontaneous regression usually occurs. In later life it must be distinguished from Hashimoto's disease by thyroid antibody estimation.

Simple goitres

Simple goitres are caused by iodine deficiency and may occur endemically or sporadically.

On palpation the *solitary* visible nodule may prove to be part of what is, in fact, a multinodular goitre (Figure 5.7). Examination of the thyroid gland, however, is not always easy.

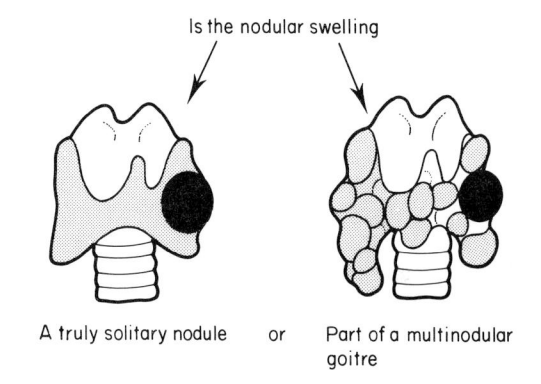

Figure 5.7 Nodular goitre.

The bilobed swelling which moves on swallowing is easily identified as thyroid glands. The retrosternal goitre or fixed gland is more difficult to identify. The anterior and posterior triangles of the neck must be palpated for enlargement of lymph nodes which may signify malignancy.

Multinodular goitre

This may be the result of iodine deficiency in the so called 'endemic goitre' or it may occur sporadically due to enzyme defects in the synthesis of thyroid hormones. In the latter case there may be a strong family history of goitre. The patient may be aware of having had a thyroid enlargement for many years, with the swelling having perhaps progressed from a diffuse 'simple' goitre in puberty to a nodular enlargement in later life.

Radioactive iodine scanning may occasionally be helpful in deciding if a goitre is multinodular.

Ultrasound scanning is now superseding radioactive imaging and may positively identify a multinodular goitre, enabling operation to be avoided in some patients.

Surgery is indicated for a multinodular goitre if malignancy cannot definitely be excluded, or for symptoms of local compression (dysphagia, stridor, deviation of the trachea on x-ray, or voice change). The size of the gland alone may justify operation.

Experience has shown that approximately 60 per cent of solitary nodules prove at operation to be part of a multinodular colloid goitre (Figure 5.7) in which other nodules were too small to be clinically detectable. This rate is likely to become much lower with improved technique of computerized tomography and ultrasound scanning.

The thyrotoxic patient

If the patient has signs or symptoms of thyrotoxicosis, a radioactive iodine uptake scan should be done. The scan might reveal a concentration of iodine in a single 'hot' nodule with suppression of the rest of the gland (Figure 5.8). Such autonomous toxic nodules are responsible for about 2 per cent of all cases of thyrotoxicosis. They can be effectively treated with radioactive iodine, but are usually best treated by surgical excision after drug control of the thryotoxicosis.

examination to be well differentiated carcinomas, and therefore surgical excision is usually advised.

Thyroid cysts

The history may be helpful in the diagnosis of thyroid cysts. Often they present as a tender swelling of sudden onset and the diagnosis of a cyst can be made with some confidence. In these circumstances it is reasonable to review the patient one month later. If complete resolution does not occur excision should be advised because 5 to 10 per cent of cysts prove to have a solid malignant component. With improved techniques, ultrasound scanning may allow exclusion of a solid component and allow more cysts to be treated by aspiration alone.

Thyroid cancer

Approximately 12 per cent of truly solitary nodules of the thyroid gland prove on histological examination to be malignant. Needle biopsy and

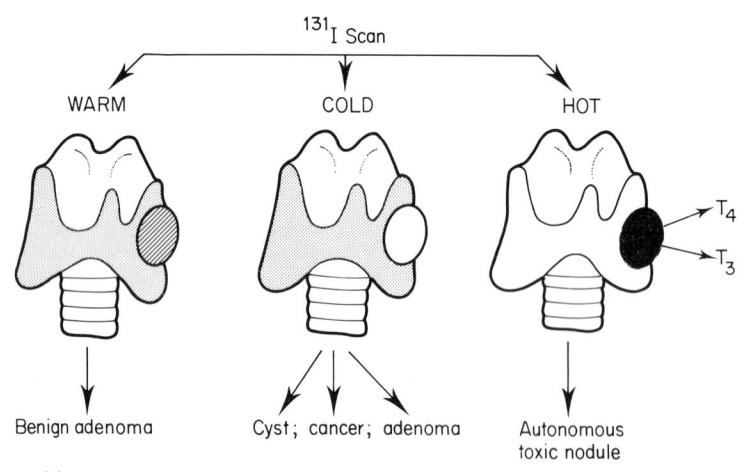

Figure 5.8 The truly solitary nodule.

The euthyroid patient

^{131}I scanning is less helpful in the diagnosis of the solitary nodule in the euthyroid patient. Cancers are classically 'cold', but cannot be distinguished from thyroid cysts and some benign adenomas which also fail to concentrate iodine (Figure 5.8).

The 'warm' nodule concentrates radioiodine but does not suppress the rest of the gland, which is clearly shown on the scan. The majority of these nodules are benign adenomas, but a small percentage (< 5 per cent) prove on histological

aspiration cytology are advocated by some surgeons for the diagnosis of thyroid malignancy. In a considerable proportion of cases however, the procedure is not diagnostic even in the hands of an experienced cytologist, and there is often difficulty in obtaining an adequate specimen on biopsy which is truly representative of the nodule. The great majority therefore should be excised for histological examination.

It must be remembered that thyroid malignancy occurs with equal frequency at any age, and thus the very young are not exempt. Benign thyroid nodules occur most frequently in the middle years of life, and it therefore follows that a nodule is more likely to be malignant in the young (Figure 5.9).

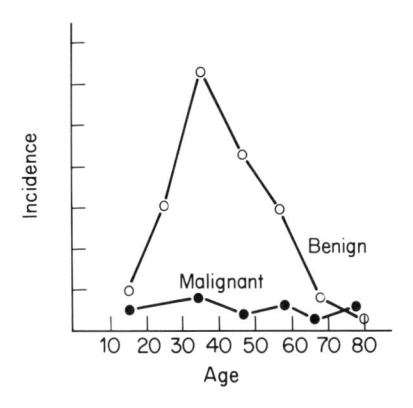

Figure 5.9 Age relationship of benign and malignant solitary nodules.

As already stated, clinical examination is unreliable in distinguishing between benign and malignant nodules. Certain points in the patient's history and examination may, however, lead to a strong suspicion of malignancy:

A previous history of irradiation to the neck especially in childhood or adolescence is highly significant, as thyroid cancers are known to follow x-ray therapy.

A recent rapid enlargement of the gland may indicate malignancy, but on the other hand it must be remembered that the doctor cannot be reassured by a long history. A papillary carcinoma may be present as a lump in the neck for several years before the patient consults the doctor.

Hoarseness of the voice due to recurrent laryngeal nerve involvement is an important clue, as is unilateral pain in the neck, sometimes referred to the ear.

Fixity of the gland occurs early, especially in anaplastic carcinoma, but this may be difficult to distinguish from some forms of thyroiditis.

As a general rule, all thyroid nodules should be referred for further investigation and if the possibility of malignancy cannot definitely be excluded, surgical excision should be advised.

Management of the thyrotoxic patient

Ideally the treatment of thyrotoxic patients should be supervised by a medical or endocrine clinic where a policy decision on the plan of treatment may be made at the first consultation. An endocrine surgeon co-operating with a general surgeon and a physician facilitates this decision. Such facilities are not always available, however, and the guidelines for choosing treatment for an individual patient are often arbitrary, depending on the expertise available and the patient's personal preference. Provided that a definite diagnosis of thyrotoxicosis, based on thyroid function tests, has been made, it is reasonable for treatment with antithyroid drugs or adrenergic blocking drugs to be commenced by the general practitioner. Arrangements must be made for the continuing monitoring of the patient's progress.

The decision can usually be made at an early stage on which of the three forms of treatment is to be preferred for a particular patient.

Surgery

This is most often the treatment choice for patients with autonomous toxic nodular goitres. Preoperative control of the thyrotoxicosis with antithyroid drugs is essential if the feared complication of a thyroid crisis is to be avoided.

Patients suffering from Graves' disease often present a more difficult problem of choice (Figure 5.11).

Drug therapy

Drug therapy

1. Beta-adrenergic blockade
2. Carbimazole
3. Propylthiouracil

54 Thyroid disorders

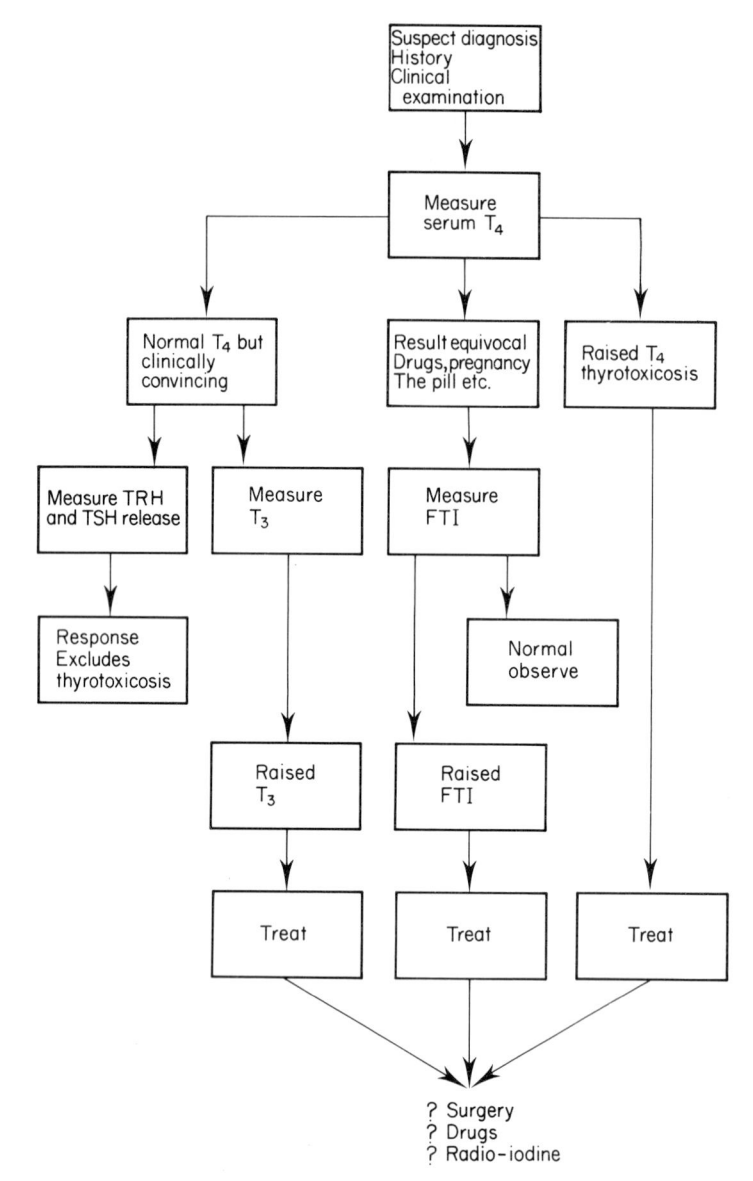

Figure 5.10 The diagnosis of hyperthyroidism.

Beta-adrenergic blockade will give rapid relief of the distressing symptoms of thyrotoxicosis, and can be prescribed with advantage in the early stages of treatment. Propranolol in a dose of 40 mg q.d.s. is suitable. Regular dosage is important because rapid return of symptoms can occur after six hours if a dose is omitted.

Carbimazole is the antithyroid drug most frequently prescribed in the UK. Its disadvantage is that a long and continuous course of treatment (12–18 months) is necessary, and even then a high relapse rate in excess of 50 per cent is seen (Figure 5.12). As yet there is no reliable indication of those patients most likely to suffer recurrence, but it has been suggested that patients with a high level of circulating thyroid antibodies (thyroid-stimulating globulins) are more susceptible.

The incidence of serious toxic side-effects is low and they are usually seen in the first three months of treatment. Agranulocytosis is the most serious, and blood counts should be done if infections such

Management of thyrotoxic patient

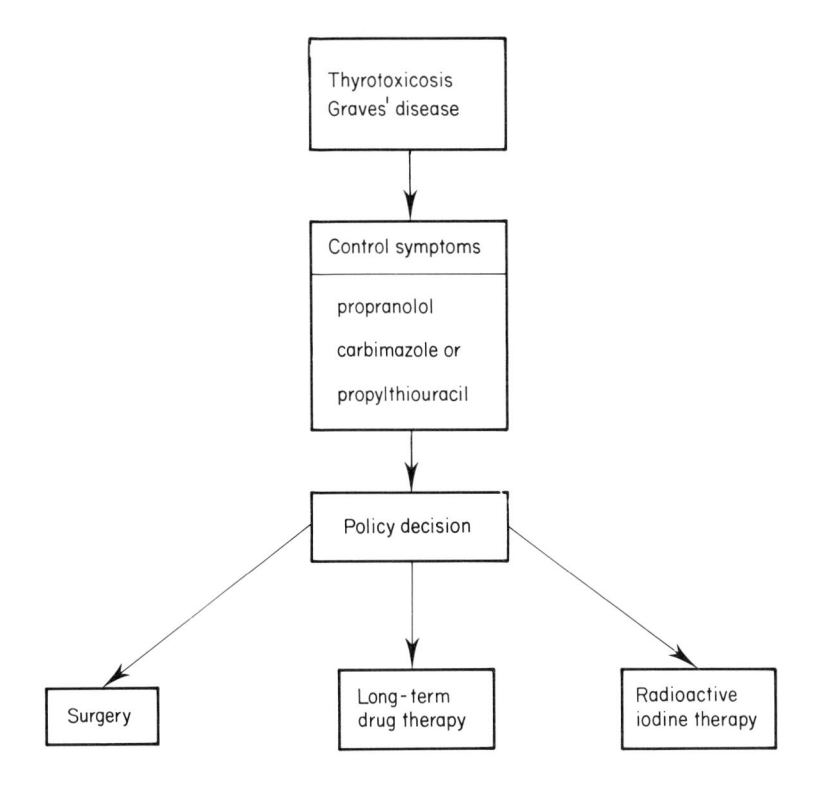

Figure 5.11 Treatment of Graves' disease.

as sore throats occur. Carbimazole is administered in a dose of 30–60 mg/day until symptoms are controlled, after which it can be reduced to a maintenance dose of 10–20 mg/day.

Propylthiouracil is used in persons who cannot tolerate carbimazole.

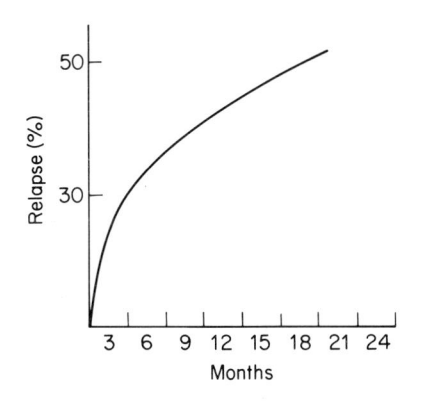

Figure 5.12 Recurrence of thyrotoxicosis after stopping drugs.

Indications for ^{131}I

Indications for ^{131}I

1. Patients over 40 years
2. Intercurrent disease
3. Relapse after operation or drugs

Radioactive iodine (^{131}I) can be used for the treatment of thyrotoxicosis, and is often preferred for the treatment of patients with intercurrent disease, or relapse after surgery or drug therapy. It may be ten or more weeks before it is fully effective, and symptoms must be controlled with carbimazole in the interval. Its use in the UK is usually confined to patients over 40 years of age because of the theoretical risk of genetic damage to those of childbearing age.

The dose of ^{131}I is difficult to judge and ensuing hypothyroidism is common: 10 per cent in two years, perhaps rising to as high as 80 per cent in 20 years. Long-term surveillance of all these patients is therefore mandatory.

Indications for surgery

> **Indications for Surgery**
> 1. Large gland
> 2. Relapse after drugs
> 3. Intolerance of drugs
> 4. Patient preference

Surgery remains the treatment of choice for many patients, especially those with large glands and those whose symptoms recur after medical treatment. All patients must be controlled with drugs if the feared complications of postoperative thyroid crisis is to be avoided.

Major complications are confined to the rare events of recurrent laryngeal nerve damage and hypoparathyroidism. The recurrence rate is low (5–10 per cent) but approximately 30 per cent become hypothyroid in ten years.

Whichever treatment is chosen, a considerable proportion of patients with treated Graves' disease will be at risk of developing further thyroid disorders at some time in their lives.

All patients with thyroid diseases should be entered into a practice 'register' to enable regular follow-up for the rest of their lives.

6 Lumps in the Breast

John Bradbeer and M. Keith Thompson

The discovery by a woman of a breast lump is a highly anxious and emotive experience. To most women, 'breast lump' = 'cancer'. It is the clinician's duty to make an accurate diagnosis as quickly as possible, in order to reassure and to treat the condition effectively.

The ratio of benign to malignant breast lumps is 3:1, and the distribution of the various types of lumps at a general surgical clinic is shown in Figure 6.1.

The annual incidence of breast lumps in the UK is approximately 120 000, of which 30 000 are cancers.

Annual deaths from breast cancer in UK are about 12 000, and the 5-year survival rate is 60 per cent.

The numbers of breast lumps that can be expected both in a general practice and at a district general hospital are shown in Tables 6.1 and 6.2.

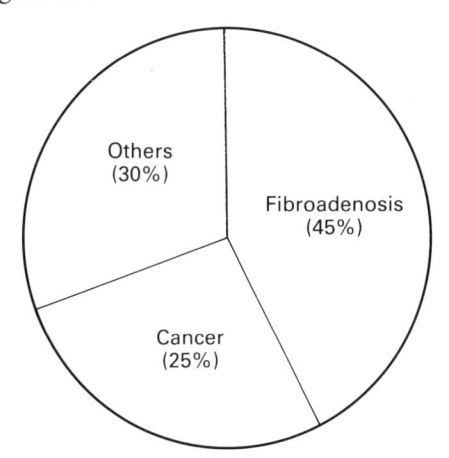

Figure 6.1 Incidence of lumps in the breast.

Pie chart:
- Fibroadenosis (45%)
- Cancer (25%)
- Others (30%)

Cause of lump	Incidence (%)
Fibroadenosis	45
Cancer	25
Cysts	15
Fibroadenoma	10
Periareolar inflammation	3
Fat necrosis	0.5
Early unilateral development ('puberty mastitis')	0.5
Other lumps associated with mammary duct ectasia, nipple discharge, inverted nipple, and Tietze's disease.	1

Table 6.1 Annual incidence of breast lumps in general practice

	General physician with 2500 patients	Group practice with 10 000 patients
Cancer	1–2 (1 death every 2 years)	4–6
Fibroadenosis	4	16
Cysts	1	4
Others	1	4
Total	7	28

Table 6.2 Annual incidence of breast lumps (estimated) per district general hospital serving 250 000.

New cancers	150
Fibroadenosis	250
Cyst and fibroadenomata	150
Others	20
Total	570

Notes (a) not all benign lumps are referred by general physicians to NHS hospital clinics.

(b) there are 4–5 general surgeons in a district general hospital. Therefore the encounter rate will be approximately 100–150 breast lumps per surgeon.

Examination of the breasts

Time of examination

Between ovulation and the onset of the period, the breasts become uncomfortable and tense. If the patient presents to the doctor with a lump in the breast at any time between ovulation and the onset of the period and there is doubt about the presence of a lump, or doubt as to whether or not a lump that is felt is of significance, the examination should be repeated four days after the end of the period; any lumpiness due to fluid retention will by then have disappeared.

Technique of examination

The patient should be seated upright, facing the doctor, undressed to the waist and in a good light. Attention is paid to:

Nipples
   for retraction or ulceration
   for variations in the level
The appearance of a lump
Skin attachment or tethering, as evidenced by dimpling of the skin
Localized discoloration of the skin
The appearance of small nodules of growth, which may be single, or may coalesce as in cancer *en cuirasse*
Peau d'orange.

Next, the arms are raised above the head. This movement may render variation in nipple level more obvious, and skin attachment or tethering will also be accentuated. The hands are pressed on the hips to contract pectoralis major. Deep attachment of a lump in the breast will be limited by this manoeuvre.

The hands are now placed on the hips, and with the patient still in the sitting position the axillary and supraclavicular glands are examined from behind and from in front, paying attention to the medial, posterior, lateral and anterior walls of the axilla.

With the patient lying supine, she now puts one arm above her head and rotates towards the midline. This manoeuvre ensures that the breast is as flat as possible on the chest wall. The breast is palpated with the flat of the fingers in each of the four quadrants. If a lump is found, the physical signs of that lump are noted: its size, shape, consistency, surface, and whether or not it is attached to skin or underlying muscle.

Fibroadenosis

This condition is also called chronic mastitis, fibrocystic disease or cystic hyperplasia. Fibroadenosis is hormone related, and occurs at any time between the onset of the periods and the menopause (Fig. 6.2). It often occurs when periods are irregular, bears a variable relation to the Pill, and recedes during pregnancy.

Symptoms

The symptoms of fibroadenosis are discomfort and sometimes pain, which is worse between ovulation and the onset of the period. The symptoms can occur in one or both breasts, and pain often radiates down the inner aspect of the upper arm during carrying and using the arm for household chores. The patient may also be aware of lumpiness or a lump in the breast. Although the symptoms usually settle after the period, they may persist for one or two cycles before regressing. There may be a gap of from three to six months before a return of the condition.

Clinical examination

Clinical examination reveals lumpiness in one or both breasts, more often in the upper, outer quadrant.

If the lumpiness is so marked that the practitioner is unable to exclude a diagnosis of carcinoma, or if there is a discrete lump, the patient should be referred for further investigations: in the case of marked diffuse lumpiness, a mammogram; and in the case of a discrete lump, for tissue diagnosis.

Premenstrual mastalgia can occur in patients with normal breasts. The treatment is the same for these patients as for those with mastalgia with lumpiness.

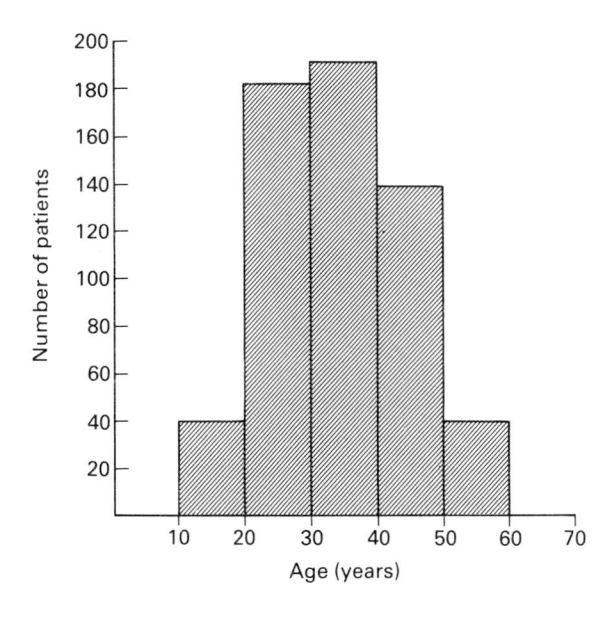

Figure 6.2 Age incidence of fibroadenosis of the breast.

Treatment

The mainstay of treatment is reassurance, and this is most rapidly and effectively carried out by the practitioner in his surgery. The patient should only be referred to hospital if the practitioner is unsure of the diagnosis, as referral to hospital induces anxiety in the patient – an anxiety compounded by the period of waiting before being seen in the clinic.

Support from a well fitting brassière is often effective, particularly in the few days before the period is due. Simple analgesics are useful in some patients, as are diuretics for four days only, once a month, if the pain becomes severe, although there is no scientific evidence to support the use of diuretics. Specific treatment with danazol in a dosage of 100–400 mg daily for three to six months is followed in many patients by resolution of the pain and nodularity. A similar response rate is found with bromocriptine 2.5 mg twice daily. Both drugs however, can be followed by side-effects such as headache and nausea.

Carcinoma

Carcinoma of the breast is the commonest cancer in women. Over 12 000 women die of breast cancer each year in the UK.

The age incidence at a surgical clinic is shown in Figure 6.3.

In England and Wales the rates per 100 000 females show different patterns.

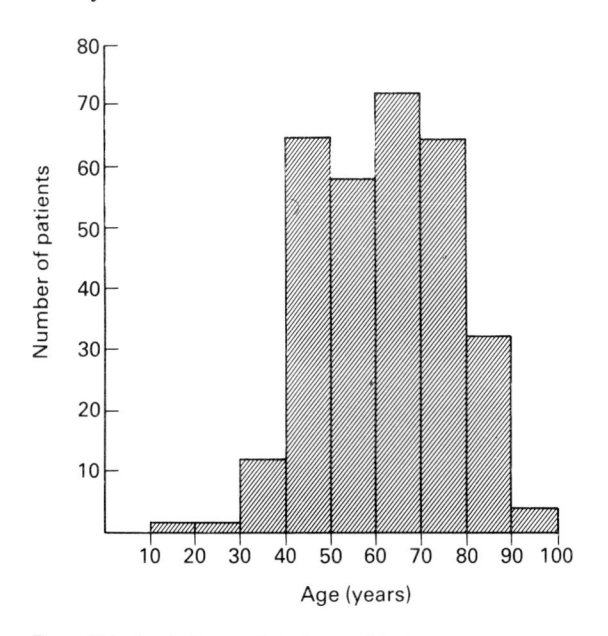

Figure 6.3 Age incidence of carcinoma of the breast.

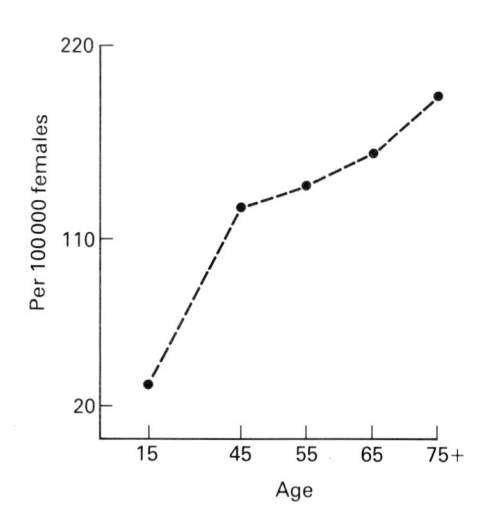

Figure 6.4 Breast carcinoma. Annual new registrations per 100 000 females in England and Wales.

Lumps in the breast

Table 6.3 Carcinoma of the breast. Annual new registrations and deaths per 100 000 females in England and Wales, 1971–4. (From *Trends in Cancer Survival in Great Britain.* (1982) London: The Cancer Research Campaign.)

Age	15–45	45–55	55–65	65–75	75+	All ages
Annual registrations of new cases	27	137	164	189	218	72
Deaths	8	67	96	121	179	39

The overall survival rates at various ages are in Table 6.4.

Table 6.4 Five-year survival rates for breast cancer. (From *Trends in Cancer Survival in Great Britain.* (1982) London: The Cancer Research Campaign.)

Age	35–45	45–55	55–65	65–75	75–85	85+	All ages
%	64	60	55	55	47	34	57

Aetiology

The cause of breast cancer is unknown. However, certain circumstances increase the incidence:

(i) Patients with pre-existing benign lesions of the breast are three times more liable to develop breast cancer, compared to patients without previous breast disease.
(ii) The chance of a patient developing breast cancer is greater if there is a strong family history of the disease.
(iii) Six per cent of patients with cancer in one breast develop it in the other.

Diagnosis

The majority of patients with breast cancer present with a lump. Very rarely, the condition can present with bony secondaries, or with Paget's disease, i.e. a malignant ulceration of the nipple due to an underlying breast cancer.

The lump in the breast is usually discovered by the patient whilst washing or drying herself. It is usually painless. On examination there is a hard, irregular lump in the breast tissue. The skin may be tethered over the lump. In the later stages the skin is attached to the lump and there may be reddening and even ulceration of the skin over the lesion.

Spread occurs to the lymphatic glands in the axilla, and later to the supraclavicular glands.

There may be a special difficulty in diagnosing carcinoma of the breast if the patient's breast is very large and also if there is nodularity in the breasts. In most instances, however, a clinician can be almost certain that a discrete, solid, hard lump in the breast is a cancer. Nevertheless there are some occasions when there is doubt about the diagnosis and thus further tests are necessary.

Needle biopsy

A core of tissue can be removed from the tumour by means of a Tru-cut needle. The skin over the lump is anaesthetized, a tiny incision is made in the skin, the trocar of the needle is inserted in the lump, the blade is pushed over the trocar, and a small hemicylindrical core of breast tumour is removed for histological examination.

Fine-needle aspiration

A 5-ml syringe with a 20 SWG needle is introduced into the tumour and constant suction applied. The needle is rotated and moved up and down in the tumour continuously in three separate planes whilst suction is continued. With this procedure it takes about two minutes to extract a satisfactory specimen. The cells are examined by a cytologist skilled in this technique.

These two techniques are very accurate in expert hands, and the method chosen depends on the expertise available. In most patients, a positive diagnosis can be made before the patient is admitted for elective operation.

Screening tests

If fine-needle aspiration or breast biopsy does not show any malignancy in a patient with a discrete solid lump in the breast, the patient should be admitted to hospital for excision biopsy, as a negative report may be inaccurate.

Mammography

In patients of cancer age, diffuse lumpiness in the breast can be so marked that the clinician cannot exclude a carcinoma on clinical examination. In these patients, fine-needle aspiration and needle biopsy are contra-indicated because of the risk of sampling error, and a mammography is thus indicated.

Mammography is not indicated in the diagnosis of a discrete lump in the breast; a tissue or cellular diagnosis is more accurate. However, in a patient with a histologically proven breast cancer, mammography is useful to ascertain whether or not the lesion is bilateral or multicentric.

Mammography can be used in the follow-up of patients with breast cancer, as 6 per cent of patients develop cancer in the opposite breast.

Staging

Before discussing elective treatment of breast cancer, it is essential to stage the disease. Screening is necessary to avoid the error of carrying out radical surgery on a patient whose disease has already spread to liver, lungs or bones.

Pre-operative assessment
Chest x-ray to assess the presence of pulmonary or pleural metastases.

Skeletal survey to assess the presence of metastases, particularly in the ribs, spine, skull, pelvis, femur and humerus.

Bone scan. Bone scanning is useful as a screen when bone pain is present and there are no overt metastases on skeletal survey.

Liver scan. There is a very small 'pick up' rate of secondary deposits on liver scan in patients in this group who are symptom free.

The main disadvantages of liver and bone scans in patients presenting with primary breast cancer are that they are expensive, and patients may have to wait some time for the tests to be carried out. An accurate history and clinical examination with particular attention to the presence of bone pain, serum alkaline phosphatase, γ-glutamyltransferase, and chest x-ray are, within one per cent, as accurate, and they are cheaper and quicker than liver and bone scans.

The site and size of the breast tumour is noted, together with the presence or absence of axillary nodes. Clinical staging of axillary nodes is inaccurate, but is adopted to allow comparisons of the results of different treatments, particularly in patients whose glands are treated conservatively.

Classification
International TNM Classification

T = *Primary tumour*
T_1 Tumour of 2 cm or less in its greatest dimension
T_2 Tumour more than 2 cm but not more than 5 cm in its greatest dimension
T_3 Tumour more than 5 cm in its greatest dimension
T_4 Tumour of any size with direct extension to chest wall or skin.

N *Regional lymph nodes*
N_0 No palpable homolateral axillary nodes
N_1 Movable homolateral axillary nodes
N_2 Homolateral axillary nodes fixed to one another or to other structures
N_3 Homolateral supraclavicular or infraclavicular nodes or oedema of the arm.

M *Metastases*
M_0 No evidence of distant metastases
M_1 Distant metastases present including skin involvement beyond the breast area.

Treatment

Breast cancer is a systemic disease and thus both local and systemic treatment may be required.

Local treatment
The main methods of surgical treatment for breast tumours up to 5 cm are as follows:

Radical mastectomy
The breast containing the tumour together with the axillary glands is removed, preserving pectoralis major muscle. Radiotherapy is not required in these patients as full axillary dissection is carried out.

Simple mastectomy with axillary-node biopsy
Radiotherapy is given to regional glands, but treatment may be delayed until the regional glands become enlarged.

Local excision of the tumour with or without dissection of the axillary lymph nodes
Radiotherapy to the remaining breast tissue is essential after this group of operations, as there is a 30 per cent risk of recurrence in the breast if no further treatment is given. Local as opposed to wide excision of the primary tumour can be supplemented by interstitial irradiation to the bed of the tumour.

Radiotherapy alone
Small tumours of 3 cm or less have been treated in France for some years by external beam radiation and interstitial radiation with outcomes as good as surgical treatment, and with much better cosmetic results.

As there is no difference in the overall survival rate following any of the above regimes, surgeons have become more conservative in their outlook and the more conservative options are gaining a greater acceptance.

Systemic therapy
It is unlikely that there will be any marked improvement in survival by the adoption of various combinations of surgery or radiotherapy in local control of the disease. Improvement in prognosis is likely to follow systemic adjuvant therapy. Adjuvant chemotherapy or hormone therapy, or a combination, have been used in many clinical trials.

Adjuvant chemotherapy with agents such as cyclophosphamide, methotrexate and fluorouracil has demonstrated a significant increase in survival but only in premenopausal women with positive axillary lymph nodes. However, there are side-effects from these drugs sufficient to interfere with the patient's life-style, and in some patients severe enough for them to stop the treatment.

Adjuvant hormone therapy with tamoxifen, an anti-oestrogen with very few side-effects, and aminoglutethimide, an agent which inhibits steroid synthesis by the adrenal and other tissues, is being used. Tamoxifen is the most promising of these agents as it has been shown to delay the disease-free interval and has recently been shown to improve overall survival in postmenopausal women.

Prognosis

The prognosis in breast cancer depends on the following:

The involvement of axillary lymph nodes
If the axillary lymph nodes are not involved the prognosis is good, and about 80 per cent of patients survive for five years. The prognosis becomes less good with axillary lymph node involvement, and the greater the number of nodes involved the worse the prognosis. Thus, with 6–10 nodes involved, the survival rate falls to 40 per cent, and to about 20 per cent when 20 nodes are involved.

Size of tumour
The larger the tumour, the worse the prognosis.

Biology of the tumour
Those patients with a more differentiated tumour and with a more marked degree of lymphocytic infiltration fare better than those whose tumour is undifferentiated.

A number of tumour markers have been assessed to help in gauging the prognosis of breast cancer, but none of them are nearly as accurate as the axillary lymph nodes status.

ER (estrogen receptor) status
In general, the prognosis is better in patients who are ER positive than in those who are ER negative.

Psychological aspects of breast cancer

Once patients are told that they have breast cancer, some are unable to grasp the fact, and in others it confirms what they thought was the probable diagnosis. Anxiety about the treatment and the future follows. Immediately after operation, many patients are slightly euphoric for a few days because the immediate crisis has passed, but this is followed in most by anxiety and depression once more. It is clear that psychological support is needed for patients with breast cancer from the start. This help can be supplied by counsellors, either lay people who have had breast cancer themselves, or by nurses who are specially trained. Such counsellors should ideally attend breast clinics. Their help is supplemented by the patient's general practitioner and the hospital doctor at follow-up clinics, as about 25 per cent of patients still have anxiety, depression and a feeling of sexual inadequacy for one or two years after operation. These symptoms are worse after mastectomy than after conservative breast surgery.

Prosthesis and reconstruction

Patients who have had a mastectomy are supplied with a temporary prosthesis before leaving hospital, and this is followed by the prescription of one of a large range of prostheses when the scar is comfortable and well healed.

Surgical reconstruction can be carried out by:

Muscle flap and prosthesis, using latissimus dorsi or rectus abdominis muscles and a silicone prosthesis;
Silicone prosthesis under the pectoralis major.

These procedures are followed by good cosmetic and psychological results and can be carried out either at mastectomy or at a later stage.

Advanced cancer

More than half the patients treated for primary breast cancer will develop metastases.

Local recurrence

Secondary deposits can occur in the skin or underlying muscle following mastectomy, or in the breast following wedge resection of the primary tumour. The secondary deposits in the skin are seen at first as small, raised, firm spots which vary in size. At a later stage, these may coalesce or ulcerate. Deposits in the muscle can be felt as hard nodules in the muscle deep to the skin flaps.

Regional recurrence

Secondary deposits may occur in the axillary or supraclavicular nodes.

Distant recurrence

The most common sites for distant metastases are the lungs and pleura, liver, bones and brain. A suspicion of lung or pleural metastases is raised because of a cough, chest pain or breathlessness. The diagnosis is made by a chest x-ray, by the tapping of an effusion with cytological examination for malignant cells, or by a pleural biopsy.

Bone pain is characterized by a persistent pain which often keeps the patient awake at night. It occurs usually in the ribs, skull, pelvis, long bones or vertebrae. The diagnosis is made by x-ray or a bone scan.

Brain secondaries should be suspected if the patient has behavioural or speech changes, or symptoms of raised intracranial pressure. The diagnosis is made by a brain scan.

Treatment

Local recurrence
Small local recurrences can be treated by excision, radiotherapy or tamoxifen.

Regional recurrence
Involvement of supraclavicular lymph nodes is best treated by radiotherapy. Axillary lymph nodes can be treated by axillary clearance or radiotherapy.

Distant recurrence
Single bone secondaries respond extremely well to radiotherapy. The pain usually disappears after one or two treatments. Secondary deposits in long bones such as the head of the femur may require internal fixation because of the risk of pathological fractures. Secondary deposits in the vertebrae may be accompanied by the risk of paraplegia and decompression of the cord may be required in addition to radiotherapy. Multiple metastases in the bones are best treated by systemic therapy.

Secondary deposits in the brain are treated by radiotherapy and systemic therapy. It may be necessary to give dexamethasone to reduce intracranial pressure.

Secondary deposits in the liver are treated by a combination of cytotoxic and hormone therapy.

Systemic treatment

Hormone manipulation
Oöphorectomy is carried out in premenopausal patients. In postmenopausal patients, tamoxifen, an anti-oestrogen which has very few side-effects, is the treatment of choice. If tamoxifen fails, then oestrogens, progestogens, androgens or anabolic steroids may be used. Patients respond well to endocrine treatment if they have a long disease-free interval or are ER positive. Those patients with a short disease-free interval or who are ER negative and with metastases in the liver or brain respond poorly. Adrenalectomy or hypophysectomy can be carried out as second-line endocrine therapy for those patients who have responded to previous endocrine therapy. Provided the patient has had a good response to previous endocrine therapy, about 30 per cent of patients can be expected to respond, although the response is only temporary.

Cytotoxic therapy
If metastases recur after, or do not respond to, endocrine therapy or radiotherapy, then cytotoxics are given. Multiple-drug regimes are followed by a better response than single-drug regimes. Many of these regimes are experimental, and patients given these drugs should always be treated as part of a randomized, controlled trial in the centres carrying out such treatment. In this way the efficacy of the drugs can be better evaluated. Commonly used drugs are cyclophosphamide,

methotrexate, 5 fluorouracil and vincristine. Up to 30 per cent of patients can be expected to show some response on the best regimes, although the response is not usually long lived.

Screening

As the results of treatment of breast cancer are relatively poor and have not changed for the last 30 years, the proposition that results should be better if the tumour is detected at a very early stage is attractive. The aim of breast screening is to detect cancer at an early, 'curable' stage. Breast screening can be carried out by self-examination or mammography.

Self-examination
Patients can be taught self-examination, and a trial of this technique of breast screening is being carried out in this country at the present time. However, compliance is only about 40 per cent.

Mammography
A randomized, controlled trial of breast screening by mammography in New York in the 1960s showed a 30 per cent improvement in survival rate in patients whose cancers were detected by screening, compared to those who presented with a lump in the breast. The results of a randomized, controlled trial recently reported from Sweden provide confirmation of the American findings. There was a 31 per cent reduction in mortality from breast cancer in a screened population of women aged 40–74 years, compared to a control group who were not screened. The screening was by a single film mammography at 2–3-year intervals. Such early detection of cancer lowers not only mortality but also the morbidity, as less radical surgical treatment is needed to treat the smaller tumours revealed by screening. Small tumours need a specialized team for excision and histological examination of the specimen.

Often these tumours are impalpable, and their detection in the breast is either by the injection of dye or the placement of a special needle in the breast tissue. The technique is carried out as follows:

The site of the lesion is assessed on a mammogram and a hook needle is placed, or a small amount of dye and contrast mixture injected, in the area of the tumour. The x-rays are repeated and a marker placed on the breast. The surgeon excises the suspicious area under general anaesthesia. The specimen is then radiographed to confirm that the correct section of breast tissue has been removed. Histological examination will reveal whether or not the excised lesion is a tumour. About 30 per cent of lesions excised in this way are found to be carcinomas. Thus, a possible disadvantage of breast screening is not radiation hazard, but that a number of unnecessary breast operations may be carried out for removal of small, benign lesions, and of some pre-invasive lesions which might not have progressed to breast cancer. However, the fact remains that the Swedish and American results show a reduction in breast cancer deaths in a screened population compared to an unscreened one.

Steroid-receptor measurement

Steroids are bound to receptor sites in breast cells as in other steroid-responsive target tissues. This ability can be measured, and the breast cancer cells can be labelled as steroid-receptor positive or negative according to their binding ability. In breast cancer, oestrogen and progesterone receptors are measured. There is a relationship between high replication rate, poor tumour differentiation and receptor negativity. Receptor status can thus be used as a prognostic factor. It is also correlated to the response to endocrine therapy. Thus, more than 90 per cent of all patients with ER negative tumours fail to respond to endocrine therapy, whereas more than half of those with ER positive tumours respond. The estimation of the ER status can be carried out either on primary breast tumour removed at initial operation, or on secondary deposits. The receptor status of a patient may therefore be of great value in planning treatment, either of the primary tumour or of the secondary deposits.

Cysts

Perimenopausal cysts

A cyst large enough to feel as a discrete lump often occurs with fibroadenosis. Indeed, the underlying pathology is common to both conditions, i.e. fibrosis, adenosis and epitheliosis causing duct obstruction. Most cysts in the breasts are premenopausal, occurring in the last five years or so before the menopause (Figure 6.5).

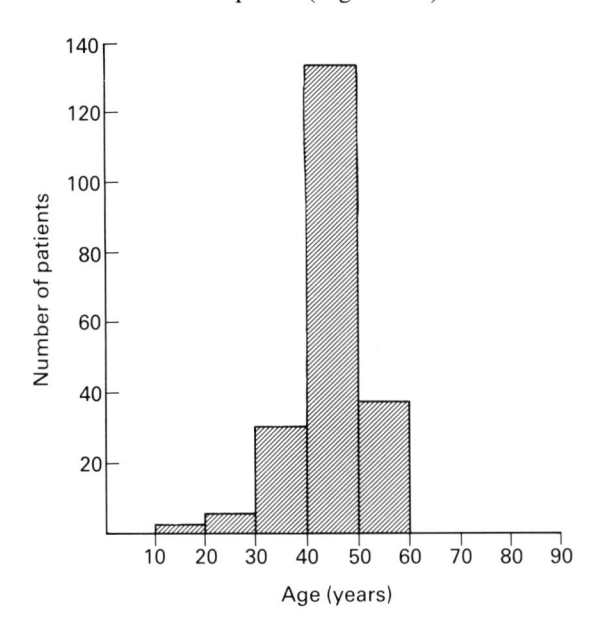

Figure 6.5 Age incidence of cysts in the breast.

Symptoms
The patient notices a lump which apparently developed overnight, often just before a period; it may be associated with discomfort and tenderness.

On examination
There is a smoth, firm swelling, sometimes fluctuant and at other times tense, which varies between one and twelve centimetres in diameter. There may be two or more cysts in either or both breasts.

Treatment
Treatment can be carried out by aspiration in the surgery, using a 10-ml syringe and a No. 1 needle. Local anaesthetic is unnecessary. The aspirated fluid may be clear, green, brown, or yellow in colour. Aspiration is safe provided that the lump disappears completely on aspiration and the fluid is not uniformly bloodstained.

Forty per cent of patients with perimenopausal breast cysts will present with a further cyst in either breast at any time until a year after the last period.

Lactation cysts

Lactation breast cysts present with the same physical signs as perimenopausal cysts. They vary from one to five centimetres in diameter and should be treated by aspiration. The aspirated fluid is usually milky in colour, but may be quite clear.

Fibroadenoma

Fibroadenoma presents most frequently in the twenties, but may occur at any age from the second to the sixth decade (Figure 6.6).

Symptoms

The patient notices a discrete lump in the breast.

On examination

A smooth, firm, mobile, usually rounded swelling in the breast is felt. Occasionally the lump is ovoid or lobulated. In West Indian patients, multiple fibroadenomata can occur, and sometimes they are extremely large.

Treatment

Fibroadenomata in the late teens and early twenties do not necessarily require excision as long

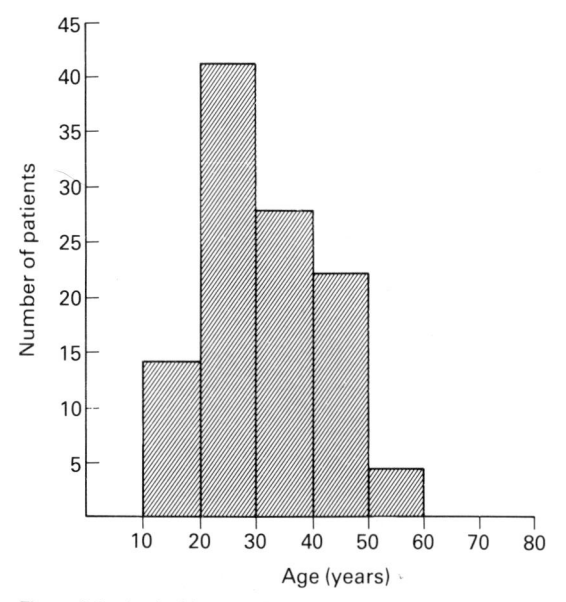

Figure 6.6 Age incidence of fibroadenoma of the breast.

as the clinician is sure of the diagnosis. The patient, however, will often indicate which treatment she prefers. A discrete lump in the breast with the clinical signs of a fibroadenoma, presenting at the age of 30 or more, should be excised, because carcinoma of the breast can mimic fibroadenoma very closely at times.

Peri-areolar inflammation

Inverted nipple
Secretion from the nipple cannot escape easily because it is inverted. As a result inflammation occurs in the terminal ducts and peri-areolar inflammation develops.

Mammary-duct ectasia
This is a perimenopausal or postmenopausal condition in which stagnation of secretions occurs in the major ducts. Stagnation predisposes to infection and leads to peri-areolar inflammation.

Symptoms
The conditions present with discomfort, leading to a throbbing pain around the areola, with reddening of the skin, tenderness, and swelling. The conditions usually respond well to tetracycline, but may take up to four weeks to resolve completely. Occasionally an abscess forms. The abscess may burst or may need incision and drainage. Healing usually follows, but occasionally a mamillary fistula between the skin and the major duct may form. A mamillary fistula will need treatment similar to that required for anal fistula: the fistulous track is laid open and allowed to heal by granulation.

Fat necrosis

This condition occurs most often after the menopause, when the breast tissue atrophies and is replaced by fat. Fat necrosis is not caused by trivial trauma, but by a severe blow to the breast sufficient to cause bruising which becomes apparent in the skin. Following such trauma, a hard lump may be felt in about two weeks, which can mimic a carcinoma of the breast even to the extent of presenting with skin attachment. If the history is consistent with fat necrosis the condition can be treated conservatively, the lump being measured at intervals until it resolves. Resolution usually takes at least two months. If there is doubt about the diagnosis, a biopsy should be carried out.

Early unilateral development

Girls as young as eight years sometimes present with tingling and swelling of one breast disc. The mother should be reassured that this is a variation of normal development and that the other breast will follow suit in a few months' time. Treatment is empirical only.

Other conditions of the breast

Nipple discharge

Patients may complain of an intermittent discharge from one or both nipples. The discharge can appear spontaneously, or only when the patient squeezes the nipple. In the latter condition the patient should be discouraged from squeezing the nipple to produce a discharge; the manoeuvre merely alarms her. Discharge from the nipple, particularly before a period, should be regarded as physiological.

Spontaneous discharge from the nipple, however, should be the subject of investigation. If there is no discharge when the patient attends the clinic, gentle massage of the breast towards the nipple may produce discharge either from one or from several ducts.

Discharge from one duct
If the discharge is from one duct only its type should be noted. A bright red colour is indicative of a duct papilloma or duct carcinoma, and the patient should be admitted for microdochectomy, i.e. excision of the duct involved. If the discharge is brown, green, or clear, a smear should be taken for cytological examination. If there is no evidence of malignant cells, then the condition can be observed; if the duct discharge persists, microdochectomy is advised.

Discharge from several ducts
This condition is associated with fibroadenosis. Discharge can be seen from several ducts and the colour of the discharge can vary from one duct to another. Surgical treatment is not indicated. The patient should be reassured regarding the diagnosis.

Breast abscess

A puerperal breast abscess is caused by infection with *Staphylococcus aureus,* which usually reaches the breast via a cracked nipple. The patient complains of pain in the breast, throbbing in character and associated with fever. The breast is swollen, red, and tender. Antibiotics given early will cure most infections at the stage of cellulitis. Once an abscess has formed, however, incision and drainage are necessary. The prescription of two or more different antibiotics, if one does not improve the condition, is to be deprecated; it will cause the formation of a chronic, thick-walled abscess.

Costochondritis

Tietze's syndrome, although not a condition of the breast, accounts for ten per cent of referrals to breast clinics. The patient complains of pain in the breast with intermittent radiation around the chest wall. The pain is not related to periods. On examination both breasts are normal, but there is marked tenderness over one or more costochondral joints. In some patients, pain radiates from the front to the back, deep to the breast, around the chest wall. There may also be tenderness over the corresponding costosternal joint.

Treatment
Reassurance regarding the nature of the condition is the first essential. It is usually self-limiting. Treatment with analgesics may help. If the condition persists, physiotherapy or a local injection of steroid and local anaesthetic may be required. If the costovertebral joints are involved, the condition could be postural and the patient should be referred to the Physical Medicine department.

Inverted nipple

Inverted nipple occurs in:
- Young women at around puberty, in one or both breasts
- Perimenopausal women, in one or both breasts
- In one breast as a result of underlying carcinoma.

History
Recent retraction of a nipple which will not evert is suggestive of an underlying breast cancer. A lump may be felt under or near the nipple in these patients, and this should be assessed by biopsy. If there is no lump, mammography is indicated. If the nipple retraction has been present for some years and the nipple everts, and particularly if it is present in both breasts, the patient can be reassured. However, the breasts should be examined in the routine manner in case there is a coexisting but not necessarily causative breast tumour. Some patients ask for treatment of an inverted nipple. Theleplasty or nipple eversion can be carried out by freeing the nipple from the underlying terminal ducts and maintaining eversion by purse-string catgut sutures. It should be pointed out that breast feeding cannot take place after this operation.

Mammary-duct ectasia

In this troublesome condition there may be repeated episodes of peri-areolar inflammation with recurrent abscesses and fistula formation. In these patients, excision of the terminal ducts is carried out by mobilizing the nipple and dissecting it free from the underlying duct or tissue, and by removal of an inverted cone of tissue that includes the ducts.

Reference
Trends in Cancer Survival in Great Britain. (1982) London: The Cancer Research Campaign.

7 The Abdomen: Acute and Chronic Disorders*

Simon Janvrin and Gillian Strube

Introduction

Disorders within the abdomen are of great importance for a number of reasons:

1. The conditions range widely, may originate in most systems of the body, and involve all medical and surgical specialties.

2. They are frequent in both general and hospital practice.

3. Potentially they may be life threatening and demand urgent action.

4. They may present difficulties in diagnosis and management, and in attempts at forecasting prognosis and outcome.

5. They provide supreme challenges to clinical acumen.

*See also Chapter 9

The roles of general practitioner and surgeon are basically similar though very different in detail.

The *general practitioner's tasks* are to make a diagnosis that may be general rather than specific, to decide on what he/she can and cannot investigate and manage, and which patients should be referred to the surgeon, and when.

The *surgeon's tasks* are to try to make as specific a diagnosis as possible, employing available modern diagnostic technologies, and to decide which cases require surgical and/or non-surgical treatment, what follow-up is required, and how best to collaborate with general practitioners.

The approach to abdominal disorders has to be practical, clinical and systematic, whether it be in general or hospital practice and a broad and practical division is into acute and chronic disorders.

The acute abdomen

The *acute abdomen* with symptoms of hours or days is a potential life-and-death condition. Although most acute abdominal conditions are not life threatening and self-limiting, others may cause death within hours unless managed correctly. Death may occur from shock, sepsis, electrolyte-fluid depletion, or haemorrhage. The acute abdomen is a condition to which urgent consideration must be given and which often demands urgent operation.

Therefore the prime rule has to be that an acute abdomen has to be *seen and examined* before dangerous conditions can be excluded. It cannot and must not be managed on the telephone or in other remote ways – and the patient may need to be seen more than once for a decision to be made.

The general practitioner's role is the most difficult, for it is he who must decide, usually on a basis of history and physical signs alone, whether the patient's condition demands urgent referral to hospital for further investigation and possible operation.

It is the general practitioner who must distinguish at an early stage relatively minor complaints such as acute gastritis (infective and alcoholic) from a perforated peptic ulcer. The colic of acute gastroenteritis has to be recognized and distinguished from early adhesion obstruction. Large-bowel obstruction may be referred too late if the symptoms are attributed to simple constipation.

What may it be?

There are many possible causes of an acute abdomen, and it is helpful to classify them:

Those abdominal conditions which may be managed at home.
Those conditions which demand urgent referral to hospital.
Those which may be due to gynaecological disorders.
Those due to pathology outside the abdomen.

Acute abdominal conditions which may be managed conservatively and treated at home (with indications for hospital referral).

Colics
 (a) biliary
   must be distinguished from cholecystitis
   may need urgent admission because of jaundice, fever or signs of spreading infection
 (b) renal
   indications for referral:
     pain ++
     fever ++

Urinary infections

 Diverticulitis
   indications for referral:
     mass
     spreading peritoneal signs
     signs of pelvic peritonitis
     obstructive features.

Acute abdominal conditions which demand immediate referral, investigation and operation

Obstructions
 N.B. signs of strangulation in volvulus and adhesion obstruction.

Ischaemia
 embolism
 thrombosis
 colonic ischaemia in the elderly

Ruptured aneurysm
 This diagnosis has to be considered.

Trauma
 This is the most difficult of all. If there is any risk of damage to organs or viscera, the patient must be referred for admission and observation.
  Danger for the G.P.: 'delayed' rupture of spleen, liver, kidney, etc.

Perforations
 peptic ulcers
 diverticular disease

Appendicitis

Acute cholecystitis
 spreading abdominal signs
 pyrexia
 jaundice

Pancreatitis

The 'gynaecological acute abdomen'
 Ectopic pregnancy
 Torsion cyst, fibroid
 Pelvic inflammatory disease.
 In all women with abdominal symptoms a gynaecological history and a pelvic examination are important.

A pathology outside the abdomen may mimic the acute abdomen and must be recognized
 Herpes zoster
 Diabetic ketoacidosis
 Myocardial infarction
 Pulmonary infections
 Torsion of testis.

How often?

An estimate of the annual prevalence of acute abdominal conditions in general and hospital practice is shown in Table 7.1

The abdomen: acute and chronic disorders

Table 7.1 Acute abdominal conditions

	General practice with 2500 patients (one GP)	District general hospital serving 250 000 persons (four surgeons)
Appendicitis	3	300
Colics (renal and biliary)	3	150
Intestinal obstructions	1	100
Peptic ulcer complications	1	100
Gynaecological	3	150
Others	> 1	100
Total	12	900

Who, what, when?

Certain conditions occur predominantly at certain times of life; knowledge of such age-prevalence patterns makes diagnosis and management most relevant.

Prevalent in young
Congenital disorders
Appendicitis
Intussusception
Torsion of testis
Henoch–Schönlein purpura
'Little belly achers'
Acute gastroenteritis.

Prevalent in adult–middle age
Appendicitis
Pyelitis
Gynaecological conditions
Crohn's disease
Colics (renal, biliary)
Pancreatitis
Peptic ulcer.

Prevalent in the elderly
Cancers
Ischaemic gut; intestinal ischaemia
Herniae
Diverticulitis
Obstructions.

What to do?

A *systematic clinical procedure* is essential. This involves:

History of present and past events
Presenting symptoms analysis
Examination.

A sensitive history and a thoughtful examination will give leads to most diagnoses and there should be no rush to resort to invasive and uncomfortable investigations without definite reasons.

- A diagnosis must be made, be it definitive or tentative
- Management – actions.

A *schematic view – site of symptoms and signs*
  RIF (Right iliac fossa) (Figure 7.1) Consider:
    appendicitis
    salpingitis
    ectopic pregnancy
    ovarian cyst
    pyelitis; kidney disease
    Crohn's disease
    cancer of caecum
    hernia.

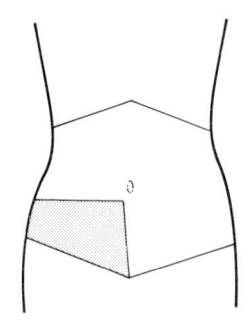

Figure 7.1 Right iliac fossa.

LIF (Left iliac fossa) (Figure 7.2) Consider:
  diverticulitis
  constipation
  colonic cancer
  ectopic pregnancy
  salpingitis
  ovarian cyst
  hernia
  pyelitis; kidney disease.

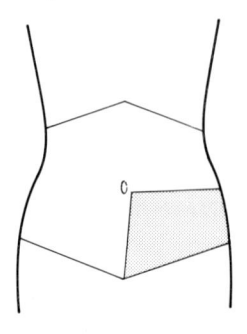

Figure 7.2 Left iliac fossa.

Epigastrium; (upper abdomen) (Figure 7.3) Consider:
- early appendicitis
- acute gastritis
- biliary colic; cholecystitis
- peptic ulcers
- pancreatitis
- liver – hepatitis; masses; congestive cardiac failure
- spleen – enlargement from various causes.

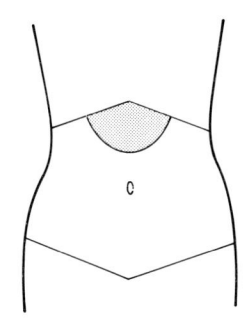

Figure 7.3 Epigastrium.

Mid-abdomen (umbilical region) (Figure 7.4) Consider:
- intestinal colics
- intestinal obstruction
- ruptured aortic aneurysm
- pancreatitis
- appendicitis.

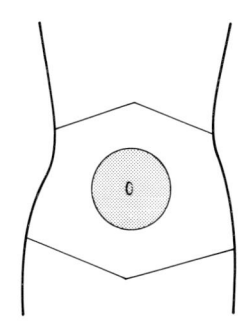

Figure 7.4 Umbilical region.

Lower central region (hypogastrium) (Figure 7.5) Consider:
- pelvic inflammatory disease (appendix, gynaecological, large gut)
- bladder.

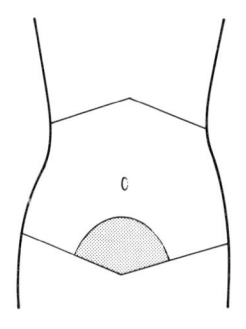

Figure 7.5 Hypogastrium.

Whole abdomen (Figure 7.6) Consider:
- spreading peritonitis
- haemorrhage.

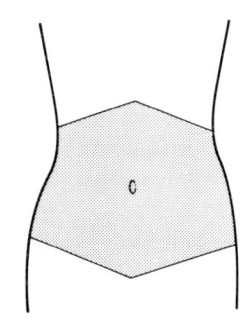

Figure 7.6 Whole abdomen.

Essential questions

The acute abdomen may present gradually as well as suddenly. The acute abdomen is a situation where physical signs demand consideration of early operation. The key to the management of these patients is not the employment of sophisticated techniques to make an accurate diagnosis, but the use of simple clinical judgement to get the *timing right*. In fact, there are only two timing decisions to be made: one by the general practitioner – '*when should the patient be* admitted?'; and one by the surgeon – *'when should the patient have a laparotomy?'*

To help make these decisions, both GP and surgeon need to consider a number of questions. A positive answer to any one may be enough to precipitate admission or laparotomy, but certainly any combination will strengthen the case for either.

Is the patient ill?

It is essential to be able to recognize how 'ill' a patient with an acute abdomen is, and it is usually something that is gained only by experience. Temperature, pulse and blood-pressure measurements are useful on their own, but repeat or serial recordings of these signs are invaluable. The pale patient with severe abdominal pain, a blood pressure of 50 mm Hg, a pulse of 130, and a pulsating abdominal mass, brooks no argument; but earlier, close observation and repeated recordings may have enabled the diagnosis to have been made at an earlier and less critical stage. A surgeon will often base his decision to open the abdomen purely on a rising temperature or pulse.

There are, however, many less tangible signs that the patient is ill. The slightly flushed face of early appendicitis, the stillness and drawn look of a perforated peptic ulcer, and the restless agony of ureteric colic are relatively late features, and the clinician has to start his assessment earlier from the end of the bed.

A manifestation of illness in a patient with an acute abdomen may be a fall in blood pressure and elevated pulse rate, signs of the clinical syndrome known commonly as shock. These signs may be accompanied by a sweating brow, pale, cold extremities and oliguria, but not invariably so in the early stages, depending on the underlying mechanism. In the acute abdomen, shock may be due to:

Blood loss
  when accompanied by pain and abdominal signs due to
    aneurysm
    ectopic pregnancy
    trauma

Dehydration in intestinal obstruction
    sunken facies
    lax skin
    oliguria

Sepsis
  Gram-negative septicaemia may accompany
    cholecyctitis; cholangitis
    appendicitis
    perforated diverticulitis.

This initial assessment can therefore begin to sift through the differential diagnosis; blood loss will tend to indicate intra-abdominal haemorrhage, dehydration points to bowel obstruction with fluid loss, and sepsis indicates perforation of some viscus.

The difficult decisions to be made early are:
  is the patient obstructed and are there any signs of strangulation?
  are there any signs of peritonitis?

Is the patient obstructed and are there any signs of strangulation?

This is a particularly difficult question in early stages in a patient with a scarred abdomen, and it may be reasonable to wait and reassess if there are no signs of peritonism. *Strangulation* must be considered if pain is severe and persistent and if there is rebound tenderness. Absence of bowel sounds is a late sign in strangulated obstruction.

Colic is the presenting sympton of obstruction, and this can almost always be elicited with careful questioning, at least in the early stage of the illness. It is often possible to watch a wave of peristalsis pass as the patient screws up his face for a few seconds whilst relating his story. In bowel obstruction vomiting comes next, but these two symptoms – vomiting and colic – are often mutually exclusive. This means that in a *high obstruction* (pylorus to jejunum), colic is often a minor feature, but vomiting is copious, leading early to 'dehydration' shock, with little or no abdominal distension. In a *low obstruction* (ileum or colon) colic is pronounced and associated with gradual distension, but vomiting tends to be late. It is important, and often appears to be poorly understood, that in bowel obstruction there are no signs of peritonism (see below) unless some complication supervenes, such as a twisted loop of bowel becoming gangrenous, or the caecum perforating due to pressure from an obstructing sigmoid carcinoma. Remember always to check *hernial* orifices in every possible case of obstruction.

Ureteric colic is the classic 'symptoms without signs' syndrome of the obstructed viscus. Although the pain is said to be 'as bad as childbirth', there are no abdominal signs, and the diagnosis has to be made on the history. The patient is never shocked, and unfortunately many a case of ruptured abdominal aneurysm has been diagnosed as ureteric colic, because the hypotension, weak pulse and pale features have been interpreted as a psychological response to pain, rather than a physiological response to blood loss.

Biliary colic is by far the commonest acute presentation of gall-bladder disease, and one that must be distinguished from cholecystitis. The former, although often more painful, is usually self-limiting and can be treated at home, whilst the latter can proceed rapidly to serious complications, and many surgeons believe it should be treated by early surgery. Biliary colic is associated with little systemic upset, and no signs of peritonism in the right upper quadrant, apart perhaps from a little tenderness. In this situation, the gallstone can confidently be expected to disimpact itself from Hartmann's pouch, with resolution of the symptoms. The signs of cholecystitis are described below.

Are there signs of peritonism (peritonitis)?

Irritation of the peritoneum by any foreign substance can cause peritonism. By tradition, peritonitis implies irritation by pus or the contents of an abdominal viscus.

Peritonism can be either local or general, and this is governed purely by the 'policing' properties of the intra-abdominal contents, particularly the greater omentum.

Any inflamed organ will cause the signs of peritonism, localized to the area of that organ; the signs of this are tenderness and guarding only. Guarding is a localized sign; generalized guarding is a precursor of rigidity, and is a sign of generalized peritonitis. Rebound tenderness is *the* sign of peritonitis, but the severe pain caused by eliciting the sign is such that it need usually be elicited once only. Thus, tenderness and guarding localized to the right iliac fossa is appendicitis, in the right hypochondrium is cholecystitis, and in the left iliac fossa is diverticulitis or the localized perforation of a tumour. This localizing of the clinical signs is the most important part of the examination in peritonism, and may require more than one visit to the bedside. Even so, almost every surgeon has been fooled by the elongated inflamed gall-bladder presenting through his appendicectomy incision, and the high retrocaecal appendix masquerading as a cholecystitis.

Localized intra-abdominal sepsis is the one condition where the general 'wellness' of the patient can belie the extent of the condition. Stoical individuals can hide a considerable amount of pus in a retrocaecal appendix abscess with only some mild tenderness and a slight fever to show for it.

Generalized peritonism implies irritation throughout the peritoneal cavity. The extent of the irritation depends mainly on the nature of the irritating substance, and to a lesser degree on the extent of contamination. In roughly increasing order of irritation are the following fluids – sterile bile (contrary to its bad reputation), blood, pus from a diverticular or appendix abscess, gastric contents, pancreatic secretions, and faeces. These substances will cause increasing rigidity and increasing 'illness', but clearly, once the diagnosis of generalized peritonitis is made, and a normal amylase has been obtained, then laparotomy is mandatory.

Some dangerous situations

- In patients on steroids, signs of an acute abdomen may be masked and minimized.
- Acute appendicitis is particularly difficult to diagnose in children under five years, during pregnancy, and in the old.
- Acute appendicitis in children may present as acute diarrhoea and vomiting.
- Strangulated femoral hernia can be missed in a fat female.
- Remember that not all acute abdomens are surgical, and consider myocardial infarction, pneumonia, pneumothorax, herpes zoster, tabes, diabetes, glaucoma, alcoholism, drug-withdrawal symptoms, psoas abscess and Munchausen's syndrome.

The chronic abdomen

The chronic abdomen typically is the patient with persistent or recurring abdominal symptoms such as pain, dyspepsia, nausea, flatulence and bowel disturbances.

As with the acute abdomen the causes of the chronic abdomen cover a wide range of possible systems and specialties.

A distinguishing feature between the acute and

chronic abdomen is that in the latter, in a large proportion of patients, no good cause can be found to explain the symptoms.

It may be necessary to accept a pseudo-diagnosis of 'chronic belly acher'.

How often?

An estimate of the annual prevalence of chronic abdominal conditions in general and hospital practice is shown in Table 7.2.

Table 7.2 Chronic abdominal conditions. Annual prevalence (varying with the age and structure of the population).

	General practice with 2500 patients (one GP)	District general hospital serving 250 000 persons (four surgeons)
No cause found ('chronic belly achers')	60	
Minor causes	20	500
Irritable bowel syndrome	15	
Gynaecological	10	150
Gastric and oesophageal	10	250
Diverticular disease	3	100
Cancers	3	300
Gall-bladder	2	50
Others	>1	100

Who, what, when?

In the young
Little belly achers
Food allergies
No cause found.

In adult – middle age
Irritable bowel syndrome (IBS)
Hiatus hernia; oesophagitis
Peptic ulcer
Crohn's disease
Alcoholism
Pancreatitis
Gall stones
Gynaecological disorders
No cause found.

In the elderly
IBS
Cancers
   stomach
   pancreas
   caecum
   colon – rectum
Diverticular disease
Intestinal ischaemia
No cause found.

'Dyspepsia'

This is a difficult symptom to unravel and pinpoint. When patients suffer from persistent gastrointestinal symptoms they use a wide range of words and phrases to describe what they feel. For instance, 'indigestion' and 'upset tummy' and 'sick' mean different things to different people. Even 'vomiting' and 'diarrhoea' often have a different meaning to the patient from that used by the doctor.

Some of the differences are cultural. For instance an Asian may use the word 'sick' to describe a general feeling of illness, whereas in the UK it is usually taken to mean vomiting. It is only to doctors that the chest extends around to the back and 'stomach' may mean anywhere between the xiphisternum and the pubic symphysis, but may usually be confined to the area around or below the umbilicus. Young children often use words like 'tummy ache' when they lack the vocabulary to describe how they feel. They are as likely to be suffering from earache or prodromal measles as from some intra-abdominal condition.

The average layman's knowledge and understanding of his own anatomy and physiology and what is likely to go wrong with it are very limited. The significance of different symptoms is also not immediately apparent to every patient. To someone from a developing country, a child with diarrhoea or a fever may be expected to be dead within 24 hours. Vomiting blood may not seem very much more urgent than passing blood per rectum to anyone except a doctor.

It is essential that the doctor makes sure that he understands what the patient means, and also that he understands what the patient thinks, or fears, he may be suffering from.

Specific causes of dyspepsia

Oesophagus and hiatus hernia

Dysphagia

Dysphagia is a gastrointestinal symptom usually best investigated first by a barium meal rather than by endoscopy. The investigation may show a benign or malignant-looking stricture, or evidence of a functional oesophageal disorder. In most cases an endoscopy is needed, and the endoscopist can proceed to dilatation-biopsy (benign) or biopsy alone (malignant), on the basis of the x-ray appearances.

- Dysphagia is one of the few symptoms that is usually clearly described: 'the food sticks about here' – and the patient points to a level usually at or above the level of the obstruction.

- Investigation of all cases of dysphagia is mandatory because carcinoma is the probable cause in the middle-aged and elderly.

- Dysphagia may be due to stricture following oesophagitis, when a long history suggestive of a hiatus hernia may be obtained.

Reflux oesophagitis

This is very common, especially in the obese and the elderly, with or without hiatus hernia.

The pain may be indistinguishable from angina, especially the atypical (Prinzmetal) variety.

The two may occur together

Both may be relieved by nitrates

Both may occur after food

Both may occur at night

Oesophagitis is often worse on bending, and is relieved by antacids.

Endoscopy and/or exercise ECG may be necessary to distinguish between them.

Oesophagitis may be a cause of persistent low-grade iron-deficiency anaemia due to repeated slight bleeding.

The symptoms of reflux oesophagitis due to a hiatus hernia can almost always be relieved medically. The number of surgical repair procedures would seem to be an indication of their lack of success. Certainly no overweight patients should ever be referred for a surgical opinion on their hiatus hernia.

Stomach and duodenum

These are the commonest sites of symptoms which doctors call 'dyspepsia', English patients call 'indigestion' and the French 'crise de foie'.

- *Gastritis* (i.e. an inflammatory condition of the gastric mucosa without ulceration) causes epigastric pain and nausea; sometimes vomiting; sometimes haematemesis

  may be due to infection (usually viral); hyperacidity; irritation, e.g. by alcohol, smoking, or drugs (aspirin or other NSAID)

  may be difficult to distinguish from peptic ulcer.

- *Peptic ulcer* is a radiological or endoscopic diagnosis. It can usually be suspected on clinical grounds alone.

  it causes persistent or recurrent epigastric pain, often with nausea and sometimes vomiting and haematemesis

  symptoms are relieved by food and antacids

  it is unwise to use H_2 receptor blocking agents without radiological or endoscopic confirmation of the diagnosis.

- *Carcinoma of the stomach* (any gastric ulcer is a carcinoma until proved otherwise by biopsy) is an insidious disease, which often has a marked geographical variation. A practitioner's index of suspicion should thus be raised or lowered depending on whether he works in a high- or low-prevalence area. However, any new upper abdominal symptoms, indigestion, or vomiting, in a middle-aged or older patient, should be investigated, preferably by endoscopy.

Gall-bladder

If investigation of patients suffering from dyspepsia reveals gallstones only one-third will be cured of their symptoms, even if the stones are removed. Whether such patients are referred for surgical opinion will depend upon their age, intercurrent conditions, the severity of symptoms, and the exclusion of other causes for the dyspepsia.

A patient with *acute cholecystitis* who develops signs of a spreading peritonitis demands urgent surgical referral because the signs may herald perforation of an empyema. The *jaundiced patient* should also be investigated early, and the presence of an ascending cholangitis may require urgent operation. In *elderly patients with gallstones* and minimal symptoms, and provided jaundice and infection are not present, a case can be made for conservative management, but the incidental finding of gallstones in the *young patient* (under 50 years) must be considered as an indication for surgical referral because of the likelihood of symptoms and problems over a prolonged period.

Pancreas – cancer and chronic pancreatitis

The diagnosis of **carcinoma of the pancreas** may be blindingly obvious or extremely difficult. One of the few things that every medical student remembers is that painless jaundice and a positive Courvoisier's sign is diagnostic of cancer of the head of the pancreas. One of the commoner features of a lesion not obstructing the bile duct is a failure of exocrine function, so any patient with vague upper abdominal symptoms and diarrhoea may have a carcinoma of the body of the pancreas. However, even with the most sophisticated of investigations this can be difficult to diagnose with certainty, although CT scanning has made examination of the pancreas easier.

The treatment of carcinoma of the pancreas, like that of the stomach, is disappointing. The jaundice can often be relieved by some type of biliary bypass procedure. This should usually be combined with a gastrojejunostomy, which will obviate the need for further surgery to relieve any later duodenal obstruction.

Pancreaticoduodenectomy is a major operation carrying high morbidity and mortality and with a low cure rate. However, it is perhaps justified in patients with small lesions in the head of the gland, or when the tumour originates in the bile duct. Chemotherapy and radiotherapy are often used, for want of anything else, but controlled trials seem to indicate that they only prolong the end by a few weeks.

Chronic pancreatitis is a rare disorder in practice. Affecting men between 30 and 50 years of age, it is usually associated with regular high alcohol consumption. The main clinical feature is dull epigastric pain passing to the back. There may be bouts of acute pain signifying acute pancreatitis. Steatorrhoea and diabetes may complicate the course.

Small-bowel inflammatory disease

Crohn's disease is the most likely small-bowel disorder that has to be considered in a 'chronic abdomen'.

A chronic granulomatous disease, it affects mainly the small bowel, but can affect any part of the gastrointestinal tract.

Clinically it may present as:

bouts of subacute obstruction
colicky diarrhoea
general illness with loss of weight, anorexia and fever
malabsorption and its results.

There may be no abnormal signs but a mass may be felt in the RIF and there may be associated perianal sepsis and anal fissures and fistulae.

Diagnosis is made on barium meal and follow-through, which shows narrowing ('string sign') of affected parts.

The cause is unknown and the course unpredictable. Treatment has to be pragmatic: surgery for complications, and various medical measures with exclusion diets, steroids, chemotherapy and management of malabsorption.

Atherosclerotic narrowing of mesenteric arteries may cause intermittent bouts of postprandial central abdominal pain. The condition sometimes culminates in acute infarction of large parts of the small intestine.

Differentiation of irritable-bowel syndrome from cancer and diverticular disease

The most fundamental question to answer in adult patients with large-bowel symptoms is: 'has he/she got a **carcinoma of the colon or rectum?**' A prime symptom of carcinoma is bleeding, and it should be assiduously searched for in patients with lower-bowel problems. The type of bleeding depends on its source. A right-sided carcinoma will bleed occultly, a left-sided lesion will have frank blood mixed in the stool, and a rectal carcinoma will produce a mush of blood, mucus and loose motion. This clearly is a simplistic view, but any hint of the above symptoms (or signs, if blood is seen in the motion at sigmoidoscopy) should lead to full investigation of the colon, and should increase the yield of early carcinomas.

A careful history will almost always differentiate between the above types of bleeding and blood from the anal canal due to lesions such as piles or a fissure. The latter is red, occurs after a normal motion, and appears on the paper, splashed around the pan, or as a steady drip at the end of defaecation. This type of bleeding, in conjunction with an anal canal lesion that would explain it, does not need a barium enema, but, conversely, the presence of piles or a fissure, and a history of bleeding from *above,* makes further investigation mandatory.

Remember that many patients attribute any rectal or anal symptoms to 'piles'. Remember too that common conditions commonly coincide.

The **irritable colon syndrome or irritable bowel syndrome (IBS)** is a diagnosis that worries clinicians because the symptoms can so closely mimic those of a carcinoma of the colon. It is not practicable to refer all patients for full investigation who present with variable bowel function, distension and abdominal discomfort. In the absence of bleeding other than from obvious haemorrhoids a therapeutic trial of a high-fibre diet is reasonable. However, it is important that persistent symptoms must be reported, and if any doubt exists the patient should be investigated.

This investigation will include sigmoidoscopy and barium enema examination (preferably in that order, as the radiologist may experience difficulty in demonstrating retrosigmoid tumours in the 'no-man's land' which is out of reach of the examining finger).

Diverticular disease will frequently be demonstrated in elderly patients with disturbed bowel function, but it must be remembered that chronic bleeding cannot be attributed to this disorder and a polyp or carcinoma may have to be excluded.

The other catch for 'barium enemas without sigmoidoscopies' are often the young patients with **proctitis.** They present with lower-rectum type bleeding, often with blood streaked on the motion, a normal rectal examination, and a normal barium enema. After all this, they are then treated with inappropriate local applications, before eventually, often a year or so later, they are referred for sigmoidoscopy, when all is revealed.

8 Herniae and Scrotal Swellings

Mark M. Orr and Brian R. McAvoy

Herniae

A hernia is the protrusion of a viscus or part of a viscus through an abnormal opening. The external abdominal hernia or 'rupture' is the commonest form and about 2 per cent of the male population have one. A hernia may be empty, or contain:

Omentum (omentocele)
Intestine – usually small bowel but occasionally large bowel (enterocele)
Appendix
Bladder
Ovary or fallopian tube } rare
Fluid (ascites).

Classification

Herniae in the groin region can be:
 Common:
  inguinal
  femoral
 Very rare:
  obturator
  interparietal
   Spigelian – alongside rectus sheath
   preperitoneal inguinal
   prevascular femoral, usually following surgery to the femoral vessels.

A sliding hernia occurs when the sigmoid colon on the left or the caecum on the right side slides down outside the peritoneum and enters the inguinal canal; occasionally a portion of the bladder may also be involved.

A 'pantaloon' or 'saddlebag' hernia is an inguinal hernia with a direct and an indirect component.

Richter's hernia is one in which only a portion of the circumference of the intestine is present in the hernial sac.

Littre's hernia is one in which the sac contains a Meckel's diverticulum.

Anatomy

Inguinal herniae can be either direct or indirect (oblique).

A direct inguinal hernia originates medial to the inferior epigastric vessels and protrudes through the posterior wall of the inguinal canal (Figure 8.1); it rarely enters the scrotum. An indirect inguinal hernia originates lateral to the inferior epigastric vessels, protrudes through the deep ring, and can traverse the whole length of the inguinal canal, eventually emerging from the superficial ring and passing into the scrotum – an inguinoscrotal hernia (Figure 8.2).

A femoral hernia protrudes though the femoral canal, which is the medial compartment of the femoral sheath, and can extend upwards in front of the inguinal ligament (Figure 8.3).

Herniae 79

An obturator hernia passes through the obturator canal in the upper lateral part of the obturator foramen in the os innominatum and can protrude into the upper medial thigh.

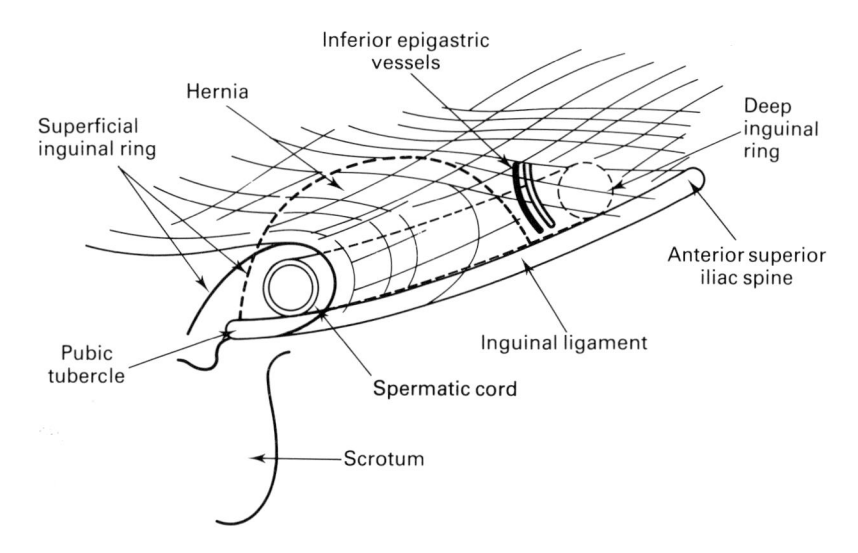

Figure 8.1 Direct inguinal hernia.

Figure 8.2 Indirect inguinal hernia.

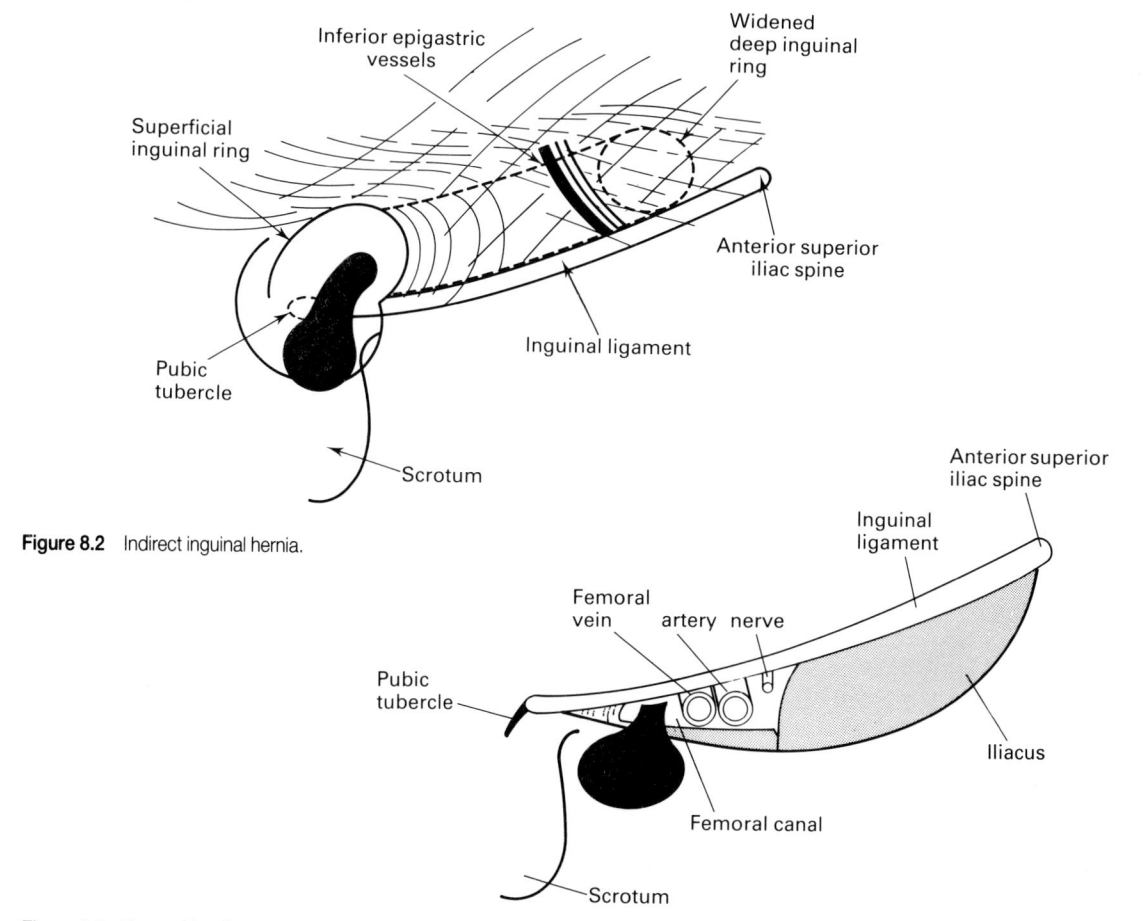

Figure 8.3 Femoral hernia.

Aetiology

Herniae may be either congenital or acquired.

Congenital herniae (See also page 8)

As the embryonic testis and spermatic cord descend into the scrotum they pass down the inguinal canal. They are accompanied by a protrusion of the peritoneum, the processus vaginalis, which normally closes off at birth. Incomplete closure or persistence of this embryological channel may result in the development of:
- varieties of indirect inguinal hernia
- a congenital hydrocele
- an infantile hydrocele
- an encysted hydrocele of the cord (rare).

These sequelae may be present at birth or develop later in life.

Acquired herniae

These result from muscular weakness, the commonest being direct inguinal and femoral herniae.

Various factors are thought to predispose to their development:

Age – they are commoner with increasing age
Obesity
Pregnancy.

In the presence of such muscle weakness precipitating factors include:

Straining, or lifting heavy objects
Chronic cough
Straining at stool (due to constipation)
Micturition difficulties (due to prostatism)
Post-appendicectomy (due to nerve damage).

A reducible hernia is one in which pressure or posture can empty the sac of its contents. An irreducible hernia is one in which this cannot be done due to the bulk of the contents, swelling of contents, or adherence to the peritoneum.

Prevalence

A general practitioner with an average list size of 2500 patients can expect to see about 15 patients per year with herniae (RCGP, OPCS 1974).

A District General Hospital serving a population of 250 000 will admit 500 patients per year for hernia operations, and the general surgeon will perform three times as many hernia repairs as varicose veins operations.

Each year in England and Wales nearly 56 000 operations are performed on inguinal herniae, and every day 8290 hospital beds are occupied by patients having such surgery. The mean waiting time for hernia surgery is just over 19 weeks, and the mean duration of hospital stay is 5–6 days (DHSS, OPCS 1984).

Inguinal herniae are the commonest type in adults, outnumbering femoral herniae by 4:1.

Most inguinal herniae are indirect (80–90 per cent), and the male:female ratio is 4:1. However, one in eight of all inguinal herniae are of the 'pantaloon' type. Thirty per cent of indirect and 55 per cent of direct herniae are bilateral. One to three per cent of all inguinal herniae are of the sliding type. They occur predominantly on the left side, and almost exclusively affect men over 40.

Femoral herniae are twice as common in women as in men, but are still less common than indirect inguinal herniae in females. They account for 20 per cent of herniae in women, 5 per cent in men, and are bilateral in 20 per cent of cases.

Obturator herniae are rare and usually affect elderly, weak and emaciated patients. The female:male ratio is 6:1.

Complications

Three main complications can arise from herniae:

Irreducibility
Intestinal obstruction
Strangulation.

All three complications are uncommon with direct inguinal herniae, due to their wide necks, but the rigid and narrow surroundings of indirect inguinal, femoral and obturator defects predispose to complications.

Irreducibility results from omentum or other contents swelling or adhering to the peritoneal lining of the sac; this predisposes to obstruction and strangulation.

Attempts to reduce such a hernia by applying manual pressure must be undertaken with the greatest care. The thigh should be flexed and internally rotated, and gentle steady pressure applied. Sudden, painful reduction raises the possibility of *'reductio en masse'* which is an indication for immediate exploratory surgery; the bowel may still be trapped or strangulated within the sac, or the sac may have ruptured allowing its contents to spread extraperitoneally.

Intestinal obstruction occurs when a portion of bowel becomes trapped within the hernia, and the narrow neck of the sac, hernial defect, or adhesions narrow the intestinal lumen. Small bowel is most commonly involved, and initially there is no interference with the blood supply to the trapped bowel. Unless the obstruction is relieved, however, strangulation eventually develops. Obstruction is suggested when a previously reducible hernia becomes irreducible and is accompanied by the following symptoms and signs:

colicky abdominal pain
vomiting
constipation and failure to pass flatus
abdominal distension
local tenderness of hernia
loss of cough impulse
high-pitched, tinkling bowel sounds.

Strangulation develops when the blood supply to the trapped bowel becomes impaired. Obstructed venous return results in congestion and oedema, which in turn leads to arterial obstruction and eventually gangrene, perforation and peritonitis. Clinically, the symptoms and signs of obstruction intensify, but as gangrene begins to develop the pain decreases – an ominous sign. A late sign of strangulation is the appearance of inflammatory changes in the skin overlying the hernia.

Incarceration is sometimes used synonymously with irreducibility or strangulation, but strictly speaking the term should be restricted to the rare situation when faeces are contained in a section of large bowel enclosed within a hernial sac.

Clinical features

All herniae present with similar symptoms, but certain features are specific to individual sites;

History

The main symptoms:

Lump
Discomfort or pain, abdominal or in the hernia itself, often described as 'dragging', and usually worse after standing or walking around, especially at the end of the day. In cases of indirect inguinal herniae pain can be referred to the testicle. In over 50 per cent of strangulated obturator herniae pain is referred along the geniculate branch of the obturator nerve to the knee.
Occasionally pain is of ilio-inguinal nerve distribution – to neck of scrotum and upper medial thigh.
Pain in testes due to obstruction and congestion of the spermatic cord (Figure 8.4, page 86)

Important points to cover in the history are:

What is the duration of the symptoms; is there any progression:
Is the lump reducible or not?
Are there any symptoms suggestive of obstruction?

Has there been previous trauma or surgery in the groin region?
What is the patient's occupation?

Examination

The patient should have both groins fully exposed and should be examined standing upright and lying flat. The general appearance should be noted – does the patient look fit or unwell? Record the weight; note the site of the swelling and whether standing up or coughing enlarges it.

Inguinal herniae emerge above and medial to the pubic tubercle, femoral herniae below and lateral to it. The direction of descent of an inguinal hernia is usually medial, following the spermatic cord; a femoral hernia tends to turn up proximally over the inguinal ligament and shows differential mobility as a result, appearing to 'swing' on the deep component. In theory, reducible direct and indirect inguinal herniae can be differentiated by applying digital pressure over the deep inguinal ring. This will control a reduced indirect hernia but not a direct one. In practice, however, this is not as straightforward as it sounds, especially in an obese patient, nor is it particularly important.

Palpation of the superficial inguinal ring by gently invaginating the index finger into the upper scrotal skin may demonstrate widening of the ring and enable one to confirm the presence of a doubtful hernia. The hernia may be palpated just inside the inguinal canal and the direction of the cough impulse may indicate indirect hernia (obliquely downward and medially) or direct hernia (straight forward).

An obturator hernia is often 'hidden' but if the hip is flexed, abducted and everted, a lump can sometimes be detected in the upper medial thigh. Vaginal examination sometimes reveals a tender swelling in the region of the obturator foramen.

Some individuals with poor lower-abdominal musculature have diffuse swelling of both inguinal regions. These are known as Malgaigne's bulgings; they are not true herniae, and do not require surgery.

It is usually possible in an adult to demonstrate a hernial bulge which has been noticed by the patient, but occasionally an indirect hernia will not readily reveal itself; this is common in children. Patients who are referred for assessment with pain *only* in the groin, do not usually show a cough impulse, although deep palpation (see above) may detect one. If it does not, these patients are best reassessed some months later.

The following checks should be carried out:

Is the hernia reducible or irreducible? If irreducible, is it tender? Check for evidence of obstruction or strangulation (see page 81).
Cough impulse not always present. Disappearance of a previously detectable cough impulse accompanies irreducibility.
Contents of herniae. Bowel gurgles on reduction; omentum does not. With bowel the first portion is more difficult to reduce than the last; the converse applies to omentum.
Abdomen and PR if symptoms present, e.g. constipation or prostatism.

In hospital a more general examination to ascertain fitness for anaesthesia would be undertaken prior to surgical treatment.

Differential diagnosis

The diagnosis of a hernia is usually straightforward, but occasionally it has to be differentiated from other swellings in the groin (Table 8.1).

Table 8.1 Differential diagnosis of a lump in the groin

Hernia – inguinal, femoral
Undescended testis
Swelling of the spermatic cord (hydrocele, lipoma)
Haematoma
Lymphadenopathy
Vascular anomalies (saphena varix, femoral artery aneurysm)
Psoas abscess
Neoplasm (lipoma is commonest)

Undescended testis – the scrotum is empty on that side.
Swellings of the spermatic cord – encysted hydrocele, usually in upper scrotum (hydrocele of canal of Nuck in females) – are transilluminable. Lipoma often not discovered until operation.
Haematoma: there is usually a history of trauma.
Lymphadenopathy. May be localized or generalized. Usually discrete and firm; may be tender if associated with infection. (See below – Neoplasms.) May be confused with femoral hernia.

Vascular anomalies:
  saphena varix: this is reducible on lying down, but has a fluid thrill and venous hum as well as a cough impulse.
  femoral aneurysm: this is pulsatile.
Psoas abscess: a rare finding but often associated with an iliac abscess and spinal changes.

'Points' in femoral triangle lateral to femoral artery.
Neoplasms: rarely lymphoma, sarcoma, or metastases from melanoma, carcinoma, or neurofibroma, or the ubiquitous lipoma can present as groin swellings.

Investigation

Most patients with herniae require no investigation – the diagnosis is entirely clinical. Patients undergoing surgery generally have a preoperative haemoglobin check; older patients may require a chest x-ray, ECG and urea and electrolyte check.

Assessment and decisions

Most patients with groin herniae should be referred to hospital. The exceptions are the very old and debilitated, but even some of these may benefit from surgery under local anaesthesia. Indeed, elective procedures carry much less risk for such patients than emergency surgery.

Patients with uncomplicated inguinal herniae can be seen non-urgently at the outpatient clinic, but priority should be given to irreducible herniae if painful or of recent onset, femoral herniae, and obturator herniae.

Obese patients should be encouraged to lose weight before referral. Weak abdominal musculature can be toned up by exercise.

Emergency admission is indicated if there is any suspicion of obstruction or strangulation. Plain abdominal x-rays may be required, but the decision to operate is usually a clinical one. Gross dehydration from vomiting should be corrected first.

Management

The mainstay of treatment is surgery, but for the few patients who decline or are too frail for any surgical intervention a truss can relieve symptoms.

A rat-tailed spring truss with perineal band to prevent slipping can control a small inguinal hernia. Patients must, however, be carefully instructed in its use. After the hernia has been reduced by the patient lying flat, the truss should be applied with the pad directly over the inguinal canal and it should be worn all day. An incorrectly placed truss pad can increase the risk of strangulation by placing additional pressure on the contents of an hernial sac.

Trusses are most suitable for asymptomatic, reducible, direct inguinal herniae in the elderly. In this small group the chances of strangulation are low and the operative mortality increases with age (Table 8.2). Trusses are contra-indicated for femoral herniae, due to the high risk of strangulation. The irreducible hernia is, by definition, not suitable for control by a truss.

A patient may be provided with a truss on a trial basis as a temporary measure to control pain pending surgical treatment.

Table 8.2 Age-related mortality for hernia repairs. From Ziffen and Hartford (1972).

Age (years)	Mortality (%) Inguinal	Femoral
< 60	0.1	1.3
60–69	0.2	0.0
70–79	1.6	2.7
> 80	3.3	6.6

Surgery

A variety of operations exist but all involve certain basic principles:

Herniotomy – excision or obliteration of the hernial sac.

Herniorrhaphy – repair of the deficiency in the abdominal wall. Usually synthetic materials are employed but sometimes fascia, skin, tendon or muscle aponeurosis can be used (hernioplasty).

Whenever possible, normal anatomy should be restored. The suture materials used (e.g. nylon, polypropylene, polydioxanone, polyglycolic acid) are matters for the surgeon's personal choice, but should be strong enough to ensure that the tissues unite soundly.

Hernia repairs can be performed under local, regional or general anaesthesia. Local or regional anaesthesia (epidural) is especially useful for the elderly or frail, but can also be used for elective surgery in younger patients. This enables the operation to be performed under day care, which is more convenient for many patients and much less expensive than hospital admission. If a long-acting local anaesthetic such as bupivacaine hydrochloride (Marcain) is employed it can reduce the need for postoperative analgesia.

General anaesthesia is indicated in emergency surgery for acute complication of herniae, and for herniotomies in children.

Inguinal herniae
The operation consists of:

Crease incision
Opening inguinal canal
Herniotomy for any indirect sac; may be merely prolapsed extraperitoneal fat
Narrowing of the deep ring – Lytle's repair with unabsorbable suture
Strengthening of the posterior wall of the canal if indicated.

In children and young adults there is no need to repair the posterior wall as a routine; its strength can be assessed with a finger passed through the neck of the hernia.

The most popular methods of repair are:

Bassini – suturing the conjoint tendon to the inguinal ligament with or without a relaxing incision (Tanner slide).
Shouldice operation – a multi-layer repair of the transversalis fascia (Glassow, 1976).
Nylon darn repair – an interlacing and interlocking nylon darn is used to strengthen the posterior wall, without approximation of the tendon and ligament to avoid tension.

In direct herniae the diffuse bulge is merely inverted by imbricating sutures. Occasionally a funicular type of direct hernia will require herniotomy, and there must always be a careful search for any indirect sac in the spermatic cord to avoid 'recurrences'.

Femoral herniae
Three approaches are available:

Low or crural approach (Lockwood). This is the most popular. It is suitable for all uncomplicated herniae, and can be extended to reduce a strangulated hernia by division of the lacunar ligament, or even the inguinal ligament.
Inguinal approach (Lothiessen). This is suitable for strangulated herniae, but weakens the posterior wall of the inguinal canal, which requires a formal repair.
High approach (McEvedy). – An extraperitoneal abdominal approach with good access to the neck of the hernia from above. It is sometimes favoured in strangulated herniae.

Whichever approach is used, the hernial defect may require enlargement to reduce its contents. It is then repaired with nylon.

Obturator herniae
Most cases are not diagnosed until laparotomy for intestinal obstruction in emaciated, elderly females, when reduction can be undertaken via the abdominal approach. These are often Richter's herniae.

Sliding herniae
This is a form of indirect inguinal hernia and is repaired accordingly. The 'sac' need not be opened, but merely reduced with its contents, unless it is strangulated (which is very rare). It is meddlesome to try to dissect the peritoneum off the colon or caecum.

Recurrent herniae
These may be technically difficult but can often be repaired by the above techniques. The recurrence is generally either indirect inguinal, or funicular direct inguinal near the pubic tubercle. It is seldom necessary to perform orchidectomy to assist closure of the inguinal canal.

Complicated herniae

If strangulation has occurred in addition to repairing the hernia, any non-viable bowel must be resected once the obstruction has been relieved.

Bilateral herniae

These are generally best repaired at separate operations. Simultaneous repairs run slightly increased risks of infection, haematoma formation, and possible recurrence.

Postoperative complications (Table 8.3)

Table 8.3 Postoperative complications

1. Bruising and haematoma; scrotal or penile swelling (particularly after bilateral repairs)
2. Infection
3. Recurrence
4. Ilio-inguinal neuralgia

- Local bruising and haematoma formation can be reduced by postoperative rest and scrotal support.
- Infection can be minimized by good surgical technique.
- Recurrence may be due to faulty surgical technique, e.g. an overlooked indirect hernial sac or a poor repair, infection, haematoma formation or excessive straining soon after operation. Recurrences are commonest within the first year. Rates of recurrence vary with the type of hernia and the repair technique used. Over a 20-year period one can expect recurrences in:

    1 in 5 direct inguinal herniae
    1 in 10 indirect inguinal herniae
    1 in 30 femoral herniae (Kidson and Britton, 1982).

- Ilio-inguinal neuralgia.

Return to work

There are no hard and fast rules about returning to work after a hernia operation. Obviously a sedentary worker can return sooner than a labourer whose work involves straining or heavy lifting. Many desk workers can get back to work within a week of surgery but more strenuous jobs may require four to six weeks' convalescence. One survey of 260 patients has shown that prolonged time off work does not reduce the incidence of recurrence after hernia repair, and also that an early return to work does not increase the risk of recurrence (Ross, 1975).

Driving can be resumed within one or two weeks of surgery, once local discomfort has subsided.

Scrotal swellings

Introduction

The scrotum is a cutaneous pouch containing the testes and lower parts of the spermatic cords, surrounded by layers of fascia and the dartos muscle. The testes are invested with tunica vaginalis derived from the peritoneal cavity during descent of the organs. The left testis generally hangs at a lower level than the right, because of its longer spermatic cord. Lymphatic drainage from the testis and epididymis passes up the spermatic cord to terminate in the aortic and para-aortic nodes. Lymphatic drainage from the skin of the scrotum passes to the superficial inguinal glands.

Classification

Disease in the scrotum may be acute or chronic, and unilateral or bilateral. Swellings may be cystic or solid or neither. The commoner conditions are shown in Table 8.4.

Occasionally a swelling may be more apparent than real, such as when one testis is absent, poorly developed or atrophied and the other seems enlarged by comparison. Alternatively, complaint

86 Herniae and scrotal swellings

is sometimes made about the small size of a normal testis by comparison with a mild contralateral hydrocele. Generally swellings in the scrotum arise from the deeper structures, i.e. testis, epididymis or coverings, rather than the skin of the scrotum.

Table 8.4 Classification of commoner scrotal swellings

Cystic	Solid	Other
Hydrocele	Epididymo-orchitis	Varicocele
Epididymal cyst	Testicular tumour	Scrotal hernia
Spermatocele	Traumatic haematocele	Oedema
Extravasation	Torsion of the testis	

Clinical features

Symptoms

Patients with scrotal conditions usually present with either pain or swelling. Pain may be acute, as in torsion or epididymo-orchitis, or chronic as in varicocele. In torsion, pain is often referred to the ipsilateral iliac fossa.

Swellings in the scrotum are commonly of gradual onset and not noticed by the patient, particularly if elderly, until they become quite prominent. The exceptions are the acute conditions of torsion, traumatic swellings and orchitis. Other symptoms include tenderness, pain on intercourse, fever (and possibly rigors) and associated urinary symptoms. Pain may be severe enough to induce vomiting or even neurogenic shock.

Signs

The scrotum is best examined under warm conditions to allow relaxation of the dartos and cremaster muscles. All contents should be assessed (Figure 8.4). Swellings may be obviously cystic and confirmed by eliciting fluctuation or demonstrating transillumination. If so, the testis should be palpated and its relationship to the cyst established. Solid lesions may involve epididymis, testis, or both but may be so tender as to make assessment difficult. Sometimes a cystic swelling is present around an enlarged testis, as in secondary hydrocele. In the absence of tenderness of the testis, firm palpation may reveal loss of normal sensation; this is a most important sign. In the case of large or high scrotal swellings an important question is: 'can one get above the swelling?' Inflammation or ulceration of the skin of the scrotum may be apparent.

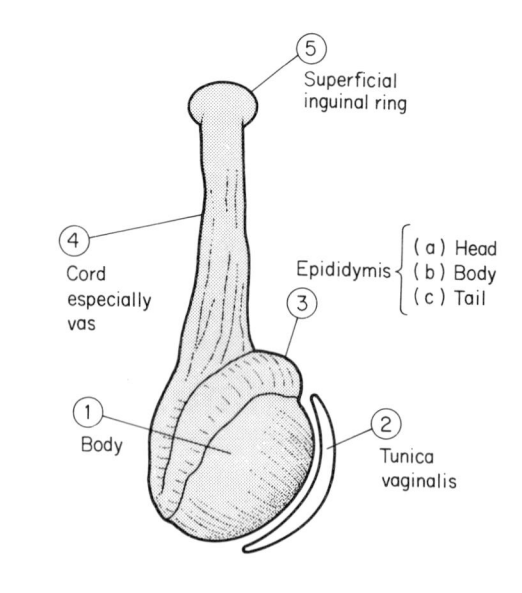

Figure 8.4 Testis in normal position.

Acute scrotal swellings

These include:

Acute orchitis or epididymitis
Testicular torsion
Torsion of an appendage
Injury.

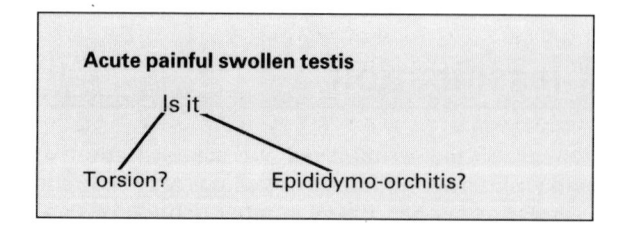

Acute painful swollen testis
Is it
Torsion?   Epididymo-orchitis?

The spontaneous sudden onset of testicular pain in a young man suggests torsion – the second most common type of surgical emergency in this age group. This may follow exercise or crossing the legs, but generally no obvious provoking cause is apparent although there is often a history of previous milder episodes. The painful swelling of acute epididymo-orchitis may follow an attack of mumps in young men, but is usually seen as a complication of prostatitis, cystitis or instrumentation of the bladder in the older age group. Thus, urinary symptoms may have been noted. Generally the scrotal wall becomes red and oedematous.

The important question is: 'can one distinguish between one condition and the other?' If not, particularly with a young man in whom a neglected torsion is a disaster, *the patient must be referred to hospital.* Unless the structure of the epididymis and the testis can be palpated individually, and the swelling and tenderness is confined to one part such as the epididymis (Figure 8.5), surgical exploration is indicated as an emergency.

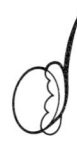

Figure 8.5 Epididymo-orchitis.

Signs of torsion

The testis is often high in the scrotum
The 'torsion' is palpable – twists in the cord or mesorchium can be felt
There may be an abnormal lie of the other testis – often transverse 'bell and clapper' type (Figure 8.6).

It is rarely possible to untwist a torsion by manipulation, but this may be attempted *in hospital* before operation is undertaken. Sometimes the condition relieves itself like previous transient torsions. Here operation is still advised. Symptoms and signs of torsion may be produced by torsion of an appendage, particularly the pedunculated hydatid of Morgagni. It is sometimes possible to make the diagnosis preoperatively, but it is always safer to operate to exclude major torsion and excise the strangulated part.

In the older age group with an atypical history

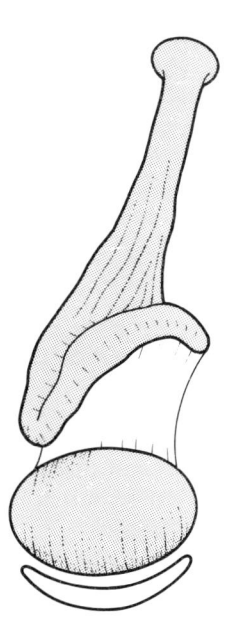

Figure 8.6 Horizontal or transverse lie of testis.

for torsion, equivocal signs, and pus cells in the urine, it is reasonable to treat as epididymo-orchitis with rest and antibiotics. The testis may be supported on a layer of strapping across the upper thighs. Generally this relieves the symptoms.

History of recurrent transient pain and swelling of testis in young man means recurrent torsion. Heed the warning and refer urgently.

Surgical treatment

The scrotum is incised over the swollen testis, and opening the tunical sac reveals bloodstained fluid and a discoloured testis with twists in the cord. Following untwisting the appearance of the testis may improve and it is best to assume viability. The testis is secured within its sac with unabsorbable sutures. The contralateral testis is always explored and orchidopexy performed if the diagnosis is confirmed. If exploration reveals orchitis rather than torsion, the testis may be incised along its anterior surface to allow decompression of the swelling; this may prevent later testicular atrophy.

Haematocele

This can be either acute, resulting from a specific injury, or an 'old clotted haematocele' arising spontaneously. The former may follow a blow to the testis or the tapping of a hydrocele. Both forms require exploration, the acute type because the testis may be ruptured and need repair to prevent pressure atrophy, and the second type to exclude a tumour. This is often impossible before the mass has been dissected, and orchidectomy should be performed if there is any doubt.

Trauma to the scrotum may produce urethral injury and extravasation of urine into the scrotum. This requires urgent operation to drain the urine from the scrotum and splint the urethra.

Fractures of the pelvis involving the pubic rami may produce much scrotal swelling from haemorrhage alone.

Varicocele

This is a varicosity of the pampiniform plexus and nearly always left sided, possibly as a result of pressure on the renal vein from the testicular artery. Very rarely a left hypernephroma may cause obstruction.

Varicocele may give rise to a nagging ache but it is usually asymptomatic. It can be seen as a bulge above the testis, which itself hangs lower down. The varicocele feels like a 'bag of worms' and with the patient standing a cough impulse will usually be felt. The varicosity empties on recumbency. In long-established cases the testis may be smaller and softer than usual, and the condition associated with impaired spermatogenesis and subfertility.

Treatment is rarely indicated – only for pain or infertility. A scrotal support or even tight-fitting underpants may be all that is required to relieve pain. Surgical treatment may be performed via a scrotal or groin incision for a direct approach to the varices, but the best technique is ligation of the testicular vein itself at the deep inguinal ring.

Cystic swellings of the scrotum

Hydroceles

These may be congenital or acquired. The commoner acquired variety may be primary, i.e. idiopathic, or secondary to some disease of the testis, usually acute or chronic epididymo-orchitis.

Vaginal hydrocele
A vaginal hydrocele consists of a collection of fluid in the tunical sac at the front and sides of the testis, and often masks it (Figure 8.7). It is the commonest type and appears in the middle-aged or elderly as a painless swelling which may enlarge to a pyriform shape. It is possible to get above a vaginal hydrocele. It may be bilateral or associated with ipsilateral inguinal hernia.

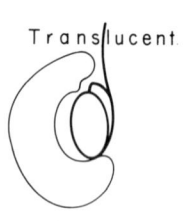

Figure 8.7 Hydrocele. (The position is reversed in anteversion of testis.)

A congenital hydrocele
This has a persistent patent processus vaginalis communicating with the peritoneal cavity. It is attended to, usually by the age of five years, by simple ligation of the processus.

Infantile hydrocele
This is similar but the processus is closed at the deep ring.

An encysted hydrocele of the cord
This is a sequestered fluid-filled segment of the processus vaginalis palpable in the upper scrotum (Figure 8.8). It will move downwards with a pull on the testis.

Hydroceles contain clear, amber fluid.

Epididymal cysts

Epididymal cysts are commonly multiple, bilateral and fairly small. They may affect any part of the epididymis but are generally found at the head (Figure 8.9). Epididymal cysts arise from cystic degeneration of various embryological remnants, including the hydatid of Morgagni. The cysts are tense.

Scrotal swellings 89

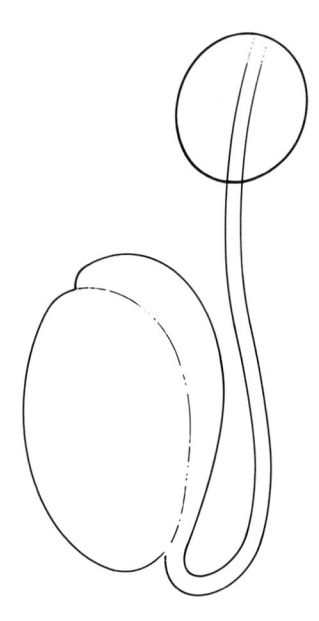

Figure 8.8 Encysted hydrocele of cord.

Spermatocele

This is usually single, less tense than an epididymal cyst, and painless. It is situated above and behind the body of the testis (Figure 8.9). When small it may be difficult to assess and transilluminate.

Epididymal cysts tend to be multiple, multilocular, and contain crystal-clear fluid. Spermatoceles are unilocular and contain a turbid fluid, like barley water, being derived from some part of the sperm-conducting mechanism.

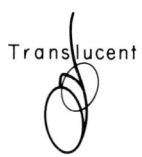

Figure 8.9 Epididymal cyst; spermatocele.

Treatment of cystic swellings

Symptomatic primary hydroceles may be treated by tapping or excision.

Tapping

Tapping, or needle aspiration, may be carried out initially with any hydrocele to help in the diagnosis and enable thorough palpation of the testis. As a means of long-term treatment it is not very satisfactory, as it needs to be repeated every few weeks or months. Sclerosants, such as aqueous phenol, may be injected to obliterate the sac but two or three injections are often required. Both treatments carry a risk of bleeding and transformation to haematocele.

Excision

This is preferred by most patients, as it is final. Excision entails opening and draining the sac, partial removal of the wall, and some eversion procedure. Jaboulay's procedure involves everting the remains of the sac and suturing it behind the epididymis. Lord's procedure uses imbricating sutures to gather the margin of the sac into a collar around the testis (Lord, 1964). As with all scrotal surgery, the patient should be warned that there will be some swelling of the scrotum post-operatively.

Secondary hydroceles are rarely large, generally allow palpation of the testis, and often subside with the underlying condition. If there is doubt about the condition of the testis, aspiration should be performed.

> If the testis is impalpable in hydrocele it is safer to aspirate and palpate.

Epididymal cysts, being multiple or multi-locular, cannot readily be aspirated. They are commonly bilateral and asymptomatic, so reassurance is often all that is needed. If they are giving trouble the cysts should be excised, and it is logical to remove the head of the epididymis to prevent further cysts forming. Spermatoceles are usually small and painless. Large or painful ones can be aspirated or may, more usually, be excised.

The smaller the size of an asymptomatic scrotal cyst, the less point there is in operating because of the inevitable postoperative swelling which may persist in some degree.

Solid scrotal swellings

These may involve the testis, the epididymis or both.

Chronic epididymo-orchitis

This is *tuberculous* in 90 per cent of cases. It may affect the tail of the organ, or the globus minor, with retrograde infection down the vas deferens from the seminal vesicle or the globus major in blood-borne spread. It is a rare condition nowadays. The clinical features are:

Testicular ache
Tender nodule in the globus minor
Firm, craggy, enlarged epididymis
Normal-feeling testis, but less mobile
Secondary hydrocele is common
Beaded vas deferens
Thickened and indurated seminal vesicle
Prostatic nodules
Cold abscess or discharging sinus in scrotum.

The majority of cases show active disease in the renal tract, or evidence of earlier disease on pyelography, and acid fast bacilli are present in the urine. Chest x-ray often shows active disease.
Treatment with full anti-tuberculous chemotherapy may not be successful, making epididymectomy or orchidectomy advisable.

Chronic non-tuberculous epididymitis

This may follow an acute attack of epididymitis and leave a painless, smooth nodule in the epididymis – generally in the tail. It does not usually require anything more than antibiotics and reassurance.

Testicular tumours

Virtually all lumps occurring in the body of the testis are malignant. They tend to occur in fit, young adults, and are of two main types – seminoma and teratoma. Teratoma usually affects an earlier age group than seminoma. The pathology is classified in Table 8.5.

The presenting features are:

Painless lump in the body of the testis – the most common feature (Figures 8.10, 8.11)

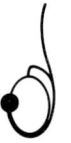

Figure 8.10 Early testicular tumour.

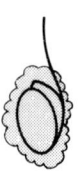

Figure 8.11 Advanced testicular neoplasm.

Loss of testicular sensation – a characteristic of this condition
Swollen testis following injury
Hydrocele ⎱
Varicocele ⎰ masking a tumour
'Orchitis'
Gynaecomastia (in teratoma)
Metastases in the abdomen, liver, chest or neck.

Each of the above testicular conditions requires referral to hospital if the findings are atypical.

Table 8.5 Classification of testicular neoplasms

Tumour	Incidence (%)
Seminoma	40
Teratoma	
differentiated – TD	
intermediate – MT1A	
undifferentiated – MT1B, MTA	32
(embryonal carcinoma)	
trophoblastic – MTT (choriocarcinoma)	
Combined seminoma and teratoma	14
Interstitial tumours – Leydig, Sertoli	1.5
Lymphoma	7
Other tumours	5.5

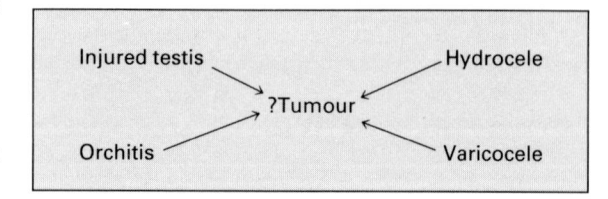

The initial step in management is orchidectomy via an inguinal incision for the first group, and exploration of the testis with a view to orchidectomy for most of the others. Usually it is quite obvious from the appearance and feel of the testis whether or not a tumour is present, but occasionally it will be necessary to open it. Frozen sections are not practicable and if there is doubt the testis should be removed. *The rule 'if in doubt take it out' is a sound approach.*

Investigations
Investigations to define the clinical stage of the disease may follow after orchidectomy. They include the following:

IVP to show mass of para-aortic nodes
Ascending lymphangiography to show nodal involvement
Tumour markers in blood – human chorionic gonadotrophin and alpha fetoprotein
Chest x-ray
CT scanning – this is occasionally useful for overall assessment.

Spread of the disease is by the lymphatics, involving firstly the para-aortic, then the mediastinal nodes, and finally the bloodstream via the thoracic duct.

Treatment
1. Orchidectomy, with high division of the spermatic cord.
2. Radiotherapy to para-aortic nodes, and later to mediastinal and supraclavicular nodes if clinical stage 2 disease develops. In North America radical abdominal-node dissection for teratoma is widely practised as an alternative to radiotherapy.
3. Combination chemotherapy in stage 3 disease, and also for trophoblastic tumours.

Results are very good in stage 1 seminoma, but poor in stage 3 at about 25 per cent five-year survival rate. The results for teratoma are consistently worse. The tumour markers help to monitor progress and recurrence.

Tumours of the epididymis are extremely rare but atypical nodules in this region are best referred to hospital.

Other scrotal swellings

Inguino-scrotal herniae may occasionally be much more apparent in the scrotum than in the groin. Careful palpation of the neck of the scrotum may reveal more bulk of tissue than should be present. Rarely a supposed testicular torsion is found at exploration to be a strangulated scrotal hernia.

> Beware the strangulated scrotal hernia presenting as a testicular torsion.

Encysted hydrocele of a scrotal hernial sac may occur due to occlusion by its contents. Following herniotomy and repair of an inguino-scrotal hernia, fluid may collect in the residual fundus of the hernial sac as this is not normally removed. It should not recur following tapping. Postoperative scrotal swelling is seen after difficult herniorrhaphies, but this soon subsides. Uniform boggy swelling is also seen in extensive peripheral oedema due to cardiac failure.

Gumma of the testis, a variety of syphilitic orchitis, is now very rare. It produces a painless enlargement with loss of sensation, and orchidectomy is indicated to rule out neoplasm.

Conditions of scrotal skin

are usually readily diagnosed. They include:

Inflammatory Fournier's gangrene. This is a rapidly progressive and destructive infective gangrene, generally with no obvious cause. If unchecked by broad-spectrum antibiotics, the process can result in sloughing of the scrotal coverings, leaving the testes exposed. Wide excision is then required to arrest the spread of infection.

Periurethral abscess and perianal (or even intersphincteric) abscess may involve the scrotum.

Sebaceous cysts are quite common in the scrotal skin. They seldom grow large enough to require excision.

Carcinoma of the scrotum Nowadays this tumour is seen in tar and whale-oil workers rather than chimney sweeps. It is usually a typical everted-edged epithelioma. Treatment is wide excision followed by block dissection of the inguinal and external iliac nodes on one or both sides.

Acknowledgement

We wish to thank Angela Chorley and Margaret Gold, Audiovisual Services, University of Leicester for Figures 8.1, 8.2 and 8.3.

References

Department of Health and Social Security, Office of Population Censuses and Surveys (1984). *Hospital Inpatient Enquiry*. Series MB4 no. 20. London: HMSO.

Glasgow, F. (1976). Short stay surgery (Shouldice technique) for repair of inguinal hernia. *Ann. Roy. Coll. Surg. Engl.*, **58**, 133.

Kidson, I.G. and Britton, B.J. (1982). Repair of groin hernias. *Update*, **24**, 195–209.

Lord, P.H. (1964). A bloodless operation for the radical cure of idiopathic hydrocoele. *Brit. J. Surg.*, **51**, 914.

Ross, A.P.J. (1975). Incidence of inguinal hernia recurrence. Effect of time off work after repair. *Ann. Roy. Coll. Surg. Engl.*, **57**, 326–328.

Royal College of General Practitioners, Office of Population Censuses and Surveys (1974). *Morbidity Statistics from General Practice: Second National Study 1970–71*. London: HMSO.

Ziffen, S.E. and Hartford, C.E. (1972). Comparative mortality for various surgical operations in older versus younger age groups. *J. Amer. Geriat. Soc.*, **20**, 485–489.

9 Jaundice*

John Bradbeer and M. Keith Thompson

Introduction

Jaundice occurs when there is excess of bilirubin (over 30 mmol/l) that is sufficient to stain the tissues, particularly skin, conjunctivae and sclera. It may be noticeable only in natural daylight.

Precise aetiological diagnosis is not easy but separation of medical from surgical jaundice is important in practice.

Epidemiology

Jaundice is not a common condition. In a general practice of 250 persons only 2–3 cases a year can be expected, and a district general hospital may admit 200 cases (Tables 9.1, 9.2).

Table 9.1 Annual numbers of cases of jaundice in general practice

	General physician with 2500 patients	Group practice with 10 000 patients
Hepatitis	1–2	6
Gallstones	1 in 3 years	1 in 2 years
Cancer of pancreas	1 in 5 years	1 in 2 years
Cirrhosis of liver	1 in 5 years	1 in 2 years
Pancreatitis	1 in 7 years	1 in 2 years
Drugs	1 in 10 years	1 in 3 years
Others	1 in 10 years	1 in 3 years
Total	2–3	10

Table 9.2 Annual admissions for jaundice in a district general hospital (medical/surgical), serving 250 000 population.

	Surgical	Medical
Hepatitis	–	100
Gallstones	30	–
Cancer of pancreas	20	–
Cirrhosis	–	20
Pancreatitis	10	5
Drugs	–	10
Others	2	3
Totals	62	138

Gallstones

Note that in the over 30s

1 in 3 of females has gallstones

1 in 5 of males has gallstones

Note that

50% of gallstones will remain 'silent'

30% of gallstones will cause colic

7% of gallstones will cause jaundice

15% of gallstones will lead to cholecystectomy

Note that in a district general hospital in a year 200 cholecystectomies will be carried out.

[Fry, J. and Sandler, G. (1986). *Disease Data Book*. Lancaster: M.T.P.]

---

*See also Chapter 7.

Physiology

Pre-hepatic

Red blood cells are broken down in the reticulo-endothelial system after a lifespan of 120 days. The released haemoglobin is split into globin and haem which, after removal of iron, is converted into bilirubin. This unconjugated bilirubin is insoluble and is carried in the blood by albumin, which prevents its excretion from the kidney.

Hepatic

The unconjugated bilirubin is taken up by the liver parenchymal cells while the albumin stays in the blood. The bilirubin undergoes conjugation within the liver cells to water-soluble bilirubin diglucuronide. The conjugated bilirubin is then excreted into fine biliary channels and passes down the biliary tree.

Post-hepatic

From the bile ducts, bilirubin passes into the gall-bladder, and finally to the small bowel. There, intestinal bacteria convert it to a group of products known collectively as stercobilinogen, which is colourless. Within the bowel, stercobilinogen is oxidized to stercobilin, which is responsible for the normal colour of stools.

Some of the stercobilinogen is absorbed in the small intestine and re-enters the blood as urobilinogen. Some of the urobilinogen is re-excreted by the liver; a small amount is excreted by the kidneys.

Pre-hepatic jaundice

The liver has a reserve capacity much larger than the amount of bilirubin it normally handles. However, increased destruction of red cells and haemolysis can cause jaundice from an excess of circulating unconjugated bilirubin. The causes are:

- Hereditary spherocytosis
- Sickle-cell anaemia
- Thalassaemia
- Glucose-6-phosphate dehydrogenase deficiency
- Acquired haemolytic anaemia
- Incompatible blood transfusion
- Malaria
- Drugs such as phenacetin, sulphonamides or para-aminosalicylate.

Hepatocellular jaundice

Disorders of the liver cells result in the failure of normal transportation of bilirubin throughout the cells, or failure of conjugation of bilirubin, or a combination of these. Hepatocellular jaundice is therefore associated with an excess of conjugated or unconjugated bilirubin or a mixture of both. It is due to:

- Acute viral hepatitis – type A or type B
- Chronic hepatitis – hepatitis-B-antigen-positive, autoimmune hepatitis, or Wilson's disease
- Cirrhosis – alcoholic or biliary
- Drugs – methyldopa, para-aminosalicylate, halothane or rifampicin

Liver tumours

In addition, there is a group of conditions in which there are abnormalities of bilirubin metabolism, and in which jaundice occurs without evidence of liver damage. The most common of these conditions is Gilbert's syndrome.

Obstructive jaundice

Jaundice may be caused by regurgitation of conjugated bilirubin back into the blood due to obstruction of the bile passages between the liver cells and the ampulla of Vater in the duodenum.

Intrahepatic obstruction

- Viral hepatitis
- Cirrhosis, which may be primary biliary cirrhosis, alcoholic cirrhosis or post-hepatitis
- Drugs such as chlorpromazine or anabolic steroids
- Hepatic tumours – primary or secondary
- Cholangitis
- Carcinoma of the hepatic ducts.

Extrahepatic obstruction of the common hepatic or common bile ducts

Gallstones

Gallstones can obstruct the hepatic, common hepatic or common bile ducts in association with stones in the gall-bladder, or as residual stones following cholecystectomy. In acute cholecystitis, oedema in the region of the neck of the gall-bladder and the lower end of the common bile duct is sufficient to produce transient jaundice, which settles as the acute inflammation subsides.

Metastatic glands in the porta hepatis
Malignant glands in the porta hepatis compress the lower end of the common bile duct. The jaundice is often accompanied by compression of the portal vein, causing portal hypertension. These glands are:

Secondary to carcinoma of the stomach, carcinoma in the region of the head of the pancreas
Primary tumours – lymphoma.

Carcinoma in the region of the head of the pancreas

Carcinoma in the head of the pancreas
Tumours of the lower end of the common bile duct, benign or malignant
Carcinoma of the ampulla of Vater
Carcinoma of the duodenum.

These conditions cause obstructive jaundice which is usually progressive. Occasionally, a carcinoma of the ampulla of Vater becomes necrotic and sloughs, allowing temporary relief in the obstruction, which recurs as the tumour enlarges.

Stricture following trauma
Eighty per cent of bile-duct strictures follow operation on the gall-bladder and bile ducts. In only 15 per cent of these operations in which trauma occurs is the damage to the bile duct noted at the time of operation.

Sclerosing cholangitis
Sclerosing cholangitis may be primary or it may be secondary to ulcerative colitis, Crohn's disease or gallstones. The bile duct is found to be thick walled with very narrow lumen. It is a gradually progressive disease lasting from four to ten years which terminates in liver failure.

Choledochus cyst
This is a congenital malformation of the bile ducts with the formation of a cyst or cystic dilatation. The condition is associated with pain, a swelling in the right hypochondrium, and intermittent jaundice.

Congenital biliary atresia
In the most common variety of this condition there is no recognizable bile-duct system. The child presents, usually but not necessarily, with progressive jaundice in the neonatal period which, if untreated, proceeds to cirrhosis and liver failure.

Parasitic infection
Hydatid disease, liver flukes or worms can cause obstruction of the ducts.

Pancreatitis
Rarely, a patient with chronic pancreatitis may become jaundiced during the course of an acute relapse.

Diagnosis

History

An accurate history is as important as the result of tests in making a diagnosis of the cause of jaundice.

Age
Physiological jaundice occurs immediately after birth but fades during the first five days. Haemolytic jaundice in the newborn can be diagnosed because nowadays all patients are screened for this condition. Other conditions producing jaundice in the neonate are biliary atresia and neonatal hepatitis. The baby should be referred to hospital to establish the diagnosis between them.

Nationality
Sickle-cell disease occurs in the coloured races, but also in some Greek, Sicilian and Turkish families. Beta thalassaemia is seen in peoples from countries in a tropical belt from the Mediterranean through the Middle to the Far East.

Family history
Enquiry should be made as to the occurrence of spherocytosis or congenital conditions such as Gilbert's syndrome or Wilson's disease.

Drugs
Enquiry should also be made into the intake of drugs as mentioned in 'Causes of jaundice' (page 94).

Alcohol

Hepatitis B
Carriers are often found amongst drug addicts or homosexuals. It should be remembered that a number of hospital personnel are hepatitis B carriers and that the virus can be transmitted by blood transfusion.

Travel abroad
Enquire into any travel in countries where hepatitis is commonly found, or there is a risk of malaria or parasitic infection.

Symptoms

Pain

Episodes of pain in the right hypochondrium or epigastrium, or across the lower part of the chest, associated with radiation to the back, should suggest the presence of gallstones. The pain may be associated with pyrexia or rigors and there may be a history of indigestion, e.g. distension after eating and discomfort after fatty food.

Carcinoma in the periampullary region, i.e. the head of the pancreas, the lower end of the common bile duct, or ampulla, are often described as painless, but in fact over half the patients with these conditions do have epigastric discomfort, and often have pain radiating to the back. A constant, dull pain in the right hypochondrium and back may be present in patients with primary or secondary liver tumours. Viral hepatitis may be painless but an ache in the right hypochondrium often occurs.

Weight loss is usually marked in patients with progressive, obstructive jaundice.

From a consideration of the physiology of bilirubin described earlier, patients with haemolytic jaundice will have a normal colour *urine* because the unconjugated bilirubin bound to albumin is not excreted in the urine. The presence of urobilinogen in the *stools* means that the stools too are normal in colour. In a patient with obstructive jaundice, the presence of conjugated, water-soluble bilirubin in the urine renders it brown in colour and the stools are pale because of the absence of stercobilinogen in the faeces.

It should be noted, however, that some patients with hepatocellular jaundice may display the clinical features of obstructive jaundice. Thus, cholestasis can be a transient feature for example in the jaundice associated with some drugs, with primary biliary cirrhosis or viral hepatitis.

The characteristics of **obstructive jaundice** are therefore pale stools, dark urine and itching.

- Obstructive jaundice will progress in patients with carcinoma of the head of the pancreas, common bile duct, or duodenum, and in patients with metastatic glands in the porta hepatis.
- It may fluctuate in patients with stones in the common bile duct, or sometimes in patients with carcinoma of the ampulla.
- It may resolve in patients with gallstones that pass through the common bile duct and in patients with an oedematous gall-bladder compressing the common bile duct, in whom the oedema resolves with treatment.

Physical signs

Jaundice
Haemolytic jaundice combined with anaemia causes a lemon-yellow coloration of the skin. In obstructive jaundice the yellow colour deepens to a mahogany shade as the bilirubin level rises.

Liver failure
Signs of liver failure are spider naevi, liver palms, finger-clubbing, gynaecomastia, testicular atrophies, ascites, bruising, and tremor. An enlarged liver with a smooth edge suggests cholestasis, as is seen in obstruction of the common bile duct by stone or by tumour. An enlarged liver with irregularly sized nodules indicates malignancy, particularly if there is gross enlargement. In cirrhosis the liver is enlarged, but the edge is firm but not markedly nodular. The liver is tender in hepatitis and also in some patients with markedly enlarged liver due to secondary deposits. The spleen is often enlarged in patients with haemolytic anaemia and in portal hypertension.

Gall-bladder
In a patient with obstructive jaundice, if the gall-bladder is palpable the jaundice is unlikely to be due to gallstones. This is Courvoisier's law, which implies that in such a patient the jaundice is due to carcinoma in the region of the head of the pancreas. It is to be noted, however, that the gall-bladder is palpable in only 60 per cent of patients with periampullary cancer.

Ascites
Ascites can be due to malignancy, portal hypertension or liver failure.

Recurrent malignant tumours can be manifest as an abdominal pain, or on rectal examination as a mass in the pouch of Douglas.

Skin
Examination of the skin may show scratch marks in patients with severe pruritus from obstructive jaundice. Needle-puncture marks are seen in patients who are drug addicts. Xanthoma in the eyes, elbows and knees occur in some patients with primary biliary cirrhosis.

Investigations

Urine and blood tests can be arranged by the practitioner and this will enable a diagnosis to be made with the patient at home. Most patients with hepatitis can be treated at home but tests for hepatitis A antibody or hepatitis B antigen should be carried out. Patients with obstructive jaundice should be referred for hospital investigation as rapidly as possible.

Blood tests

Serum bilirubin
The laboratory assays total bilirubin, but can measure its two components, conjugated and unconjugated bilirubin. The relative amount of unconjugated bilirubin is high in haemolytic jaundice, while conjugated bilirubin is high in obstructive jaundice. The unconjugated bilirubin is raised in Gilbert's syndrome.

The presence of jaundice is confirmed if the total serum bilirubin is above 30 mmol/l.

Proteins
In chronic liver disease the serum albumin is low. Blood should always be taken without stasis for this investigation. (Release the tourniquet before taking the blood.)

Serum alkaline phosphatase
In obstructive jaundice the serum alkaline phosphatase is usually very high. It is normal in haemolytic jaundice, but may be raised in hepatocellular jaundice.

Transaminase
Transaminases, liver-cell enzymes, are high in hepatocellular jaundice, and may be above normal in cholestatic jaundice. There is a typical pattern of these transaminases: with hepatitis or inflammatory conditions which are reversible, the ALT is higher than the AST. Where there is cell death, as in cirrhosis or metastases to the liver, the AST is higher than the ALT.

A full blood count
This must be carried out because haemolysis will cause anaemia. Spherocytosis will be seen on a film, and in a diagnosis of haemolytic anaemia it can be verified by red-cell fragility, Coombs' test, and reticulocytosis.

Hepatitis B antigen
This is positive in acute hepatitis B infection, and in carriers. Hepatitis A antibody is high in patients with recent viral hepatitis, but about 50 per cent of the population over the age of 50 have a positive test.

Prothrombin time
In obstructive or hepatocellular jaundice the prothrombin time is corrected by the administration of vitamin K, and this is essential before carrying out investigations such as percutaneous transhepatic cholangiography, endoscopic radiological retrograde cholangio-pancreatography (ERCP), liver biopsy, and elective surgery. The prothrombin time is normal in haemolytic anaemia.

Urine

The presence of bilirubin (regurgitated conjugated bilirubin) in the urine is always pathological. Urobilinogen, on the other hand, is a normal constituent of urine and its absence means complete obstruction.

Increased urobilinogen (in haemolytic jaundice) can only be measured in timed collections of urine, and is therefore difficult to assess. 'Increased urobilinogen' is often incorrectly said to be present when a patient is dehydrated and the urine concentrated.

Faeces

In biliary obstruction, there is an absence of bile pigment so that the faeces are pale. A positive occult blood suggests a carcinoma in the region of the ampulla or the duodenum, or bleeding from the oesophageal varices, or a neoplasm elsewhere in the alimentary tract.

Ultrasound

An ultrasound scan will demonstrate dilatation of the bile ducts, both intra- and extrahepatic, together with the level of the obstruction. The obstructing lesion, whether stone, stricture or neoplasm, can be demonstrated together with the presence or absence of disease in the liver, pancreas, gall-bladder or porta hepatis. The advantage of this technique is that it is non-invasive. Fine-needle aspiration of a tumour can be carried out in conjunction with ultrasound. However, the amount of information gained depends on the skill of the radiologist carrying out the investigation. If the ultrasound fails to display dilatation of the bile ducts, the assumption is that the jaundice is not cholestatic and therefore, a liver scan and a liver biopsy are indicated to elucidate the cause. The commonest causes of jaundice in these circumstances are cirrhosis or secondary tumours of the liver.

Computer-assisted tomography

A CAT scan will define obstruction of the intra- and extrahepatic ducts in the liver, and the site and size of the obstructing lesion. It is possible to carry out a fine-needle biopsy of the obstructing lesion, which can be useful if the obstruction is a carcinoma in the region of the head of the pancreas. As there are fewer CAT scan than ultrasound facilities, there is usually a delay in most hospitals before this investigation can be carried out.

Percutaneous transhepatic cholangiography

If ultrasound shows dilatation of the bile ducts but the exact cause cannot be defined, PTC can be carried out. After checking that the prothrombin time is normal, a fine, flexible (Chiba) needle is inserted into the liver under local anaesthetic. The needle is manoeuvred into a dilated bile duct, and the positioning is checked by aspiration of bile from the needle. Contrast medium is injected into the dilated duct. The dye demonstrates the dilated ducts, the site of obstruction, and the cause of the obstruction. A fine catheter can be left in the duct to drain the liver if necessary. Continuous drainage of bile decompresses the liver and attenuates the jaundice. This technique has been used to reduce the degree of jaundice before surgical treatment of an obstructing lesion. However, it carries a risk of infection of the ducts, cholangitis, and possible septicaemia.

In patients with inoperable obstruction of the bile ducts due to carcinoma or compression of the common bile duct by malignant glands in the porta hepatis, a plastic tube prosthesis can be introduced through the obstruction, using the transhepatic approach. Following intubation of a dilated duct, a fine wire is passed through the obstruction and a plastic tube prosthesis threaded over the wire through the obstruction. The guide-wire is then removed, leaving the prosthesis in situ.

The risks of PTC are higher than those of ultrasound because there is a very slight possibility of leakage of bile from the liver at the site of insertion of the needle.

Pancreatic arteriogram

A catheter passed via the femoral artery can be used to cannulate the pancreatic vessels so that a pancreatic arteriogram can be carried out. This examination is particularly useful in distinguishing pancreatitis from a carcinoma in the region of the head of the pancreas, as the blood-vessel pattern will be normal in pancreatitis. The procedure will accurately define the site and size of a tumour in the region of the head of the pancreas.

Oral gastroduodenoscopy (OGD)

OGD will delineate a cancer of the ampulla of Vater or a primary carcinoma of the duodenum. A biopsy of the lesion can be carried out at the same time.

ERCP

A side-viewing endoscope is passed into the duodenum and a catheter is passed via the endoscope into the duodenal papilla. Contrast medium can be injected into the common bile duct or the pancreatic duct to delineate the obstructing lesion.

The hazards of ERCP are sepsis and pancreatitis, which occur in about one per cent of patients. Sepsis occurs particularly in patients with infected bile or cholestasis. In the investigation of obstructive jaundice with dilated bile ducts, the increased sensitivity of ultrasound examinations has superseded ERCP in this particular field.

The choice of investigation depends on the expertise available at the hospital to which the patient is referred.

Surgical treatment

Preoperatively

The *risks of operating* on a patient with obstructive jaundice are bleeding, renal failure, and sepsis.

Bleeding
Patients with biliary obstruction are unable to absorb the fat-soluble vitamin K. Prothrombin deficiency results in prolonged prothrombin time and this increases bleeding during operation. Vitamin K depletion can be corrected by giving the water-soluble menadiol sodium diphosphate (Synkavit) 10 mg daily by mouth or by injection until the prothrombin time returns to normal.

Renal failure
Patients undergoing operation for obstructive jaundice are at risk from renal failure due to a low glomerular filtration rate and endotoxaemia.

A low glomerular filtration rate. It is very important that these patients are well hydrated before coming to theatre and a 5 per cent dextrose solution is given intravenously for eight hours before operation. At the commencement of the anaesthetic, 100 ml of 10 per cent mannitol is given intravenously to produce diuresis during the course of operation and minimize the risk of renal shut down. The urine output and fluid balance are carefully checked in the postoperative period.

Endotoxins. It has been suggested that in jaundiced patients there is a failure of the liver to remove endotoxins from the portal venous blood. The resulting endotoxaemia may be one of the reasons for a change in renal function, contributing to renal failure. Preoperative sterilization of the bowel to reduce the production of endotoxins may therefore be of value in these patients.

Sepsis
In patients with cholestasis, bowel organisms are often present in the bile. Routine antibiotic prophylaxis is indicated to prevent cholangitis and possible bacteraemia.

Treatment of obstructive jaundice

Until recently the correction of obstructive jaundice has been surgical. With the development of techniques such as retrieval of stones from the common duct by endoscopic techniques and the passage of tubes either endoscopically or transhepatically through biliary-duct growths, the value of surgical treatment in some conditions is under review.

Stones in the common bile duct

Stones in the common bile duct following cholecystectomy are not uncommon and occur despite the most expert surgery. At operation the presence of these residual stones is confirmed by cholangiography or by choledochoscopy. The stones are removed by opening the duct above the duodenum, or by opening the duodenum and removing the stones after dividing the sphincter at the lower end of the common bile duct. If a stone is impacted in the lower end of the common bile duct or if there is doubt regarding the complete removal of stones, then the surgeon can carry out a choledochoduodenostomy, i.e. an anastomosis between the common bile duct and the duodenum. This operation allows the bile to bypass the lower end of the common bile duct and prevents further episodes of bile-duct obstruction.

Reoperation in the region of the lower end of the common bile duct can be technically difficult and may cause an increase in postoperative morbidity and mortality. An alternative method to operation in these patients is to carry out a sphincterotomy and to remove the stones via a fibreoptic endoscope. The endoscope is passed into the duodenum, a small knife is used to enlarge the sphincter, and an instrument is passed up into the common bile duct which then extracts the stones. Removal of stones in this manner probably carries less risk than operation, especially in patients who have had multiple operations on the bile ducts, or in poor-risk patients with cardiac or respiratory disease. Endoscopic removal of stones is not entirely without risk: it can be followed by sepsis, by bleeding, or by pancreatitis.

Traumatic stricture

Stricture of the common bile duct following cholecystectomy is fortunately uncommon. However 90 per cent of biliary strictures follow cholangitis, and in only 15 per cent of patients who develop a stricture is the change noticed at the time of cholecystectomy. Reconstruction is carried out by anastomosing a loop of small bowel to normal duct tissue above the stricture, choledochojejunostomy.

Carcinoma in the region of the ampulla, the lower end of the common bile duct, and the head of the pancreas

Carcinoma of the ampulla of Vater, because the lesion tends to grow into the duodenum rather than into the pancreas, can often be successfully removed. If the lesion is very small it can be removed by diathermy excision after opening the duodenum. If the lesion is more than 1.5 cm in diameter, a pancreaticoduodenectomy (Whipple's operation) is indicated. The prognosis in these patients is poor.

Carcinoma at the lower end of the common bile duct, or in the head of the pancreas, however, present very late, and in only 10 per cent of patients is it possible to find and resect a tumour of less than 3 cm. If the preoperative tests show such a small tumour and it is confirmed at operation by Tru-cut biopsy, a Whipple's operation carries a low mortality and the patients survive longer than after a bypass operation. If the tumour is larger than 3 cm or is attached to the inferior mesenteric vein, a Whipple's operation should not be attempted, as in these patients, mortality following such an operation is about 20 per cent. These patients are treated by choledochojejunostomy to bypass the obstruction at the lower end of the common bile duct, and because at a later stage the tumour will tend to obstruct the duodenum, a gastrojejunostomy is also carried out. If the tumour is not resectable in this group of patients, endoscopic intubation can be carried out, and it is possible that intubation of the growth may carry a lower mortality than a surgical bypass operation.

Carcinoma of the hepatic or common hepatic ducts

This can be treated by excision or a plastic prosthesis.

Excision. In a few patients, these tumours are resectable. An anastomosis between small bowel and normal duct above the tumour is performed.

A plastic prosthesis is passed via the transhepatic route through the obstructed lesion. An iridium wire is then passed into the prosthesis by the same route to irradiate the tumour.

Sclerosing cholangitis

Progressive inflammatory disease of the common bile duct is an uncommon condition, but a difficult one to treat. Antibiotics and steroids have been used with but limited success. The condition usually ends in liver failure after four to ten years.

Secondary deposits obstructing the common bile duct

Jaundice due to pressure on the common bile duct by secondary deposits can be relieved temporarily by a stent passed by percutaneous transhepatic or endoscopic routes.

Commonest causes of obstructive jaundice

Gallstones

Metastases in porta hepatis

Carcinoma of the pancreas

10 Low Back Pain

Timothy Morley and John Fry

Low back pain has an enormous impact on Western Society. At least 80 per cent of the population have back trouble at some time in their lives (Auchinloss 1983). Paradoxically, despite the fact that much time and energy is devoted to the diagnosis and treatment of back pain, it causes a much greater problem in the developed quarter of the world, the rest of mankind managing very well despite the lack of modern diagnostic facilities, treatment and surgery, and also perhaps, more importantly, without any form of social security.

It is hardly surprising that the spine is a source of so many problems when one considers that the body weight is transmitted along the bony skeleton supported by its associated ligaments and muscles. Add to this the stresses of a bipedal way of life and the insults of trauma, lifting and carrying, and twisting and turning, and it is hardly surprising that the back is prone to biomechanical failure.

Facts and figures *(Back Pain, 1985)*

Together with respiratory disease, heart trouble, arthritis and rheumatism, backache is one of the commonest causes of morbidity, particularly in the middle years of life in the U.K.

Back pain represents 2.6 per cent of the general practice workload.
One million patients consult their general practitioner annually for back pain.
Fifteen per cent are referred for specialist opinion – 330 000 referrals.
Twenty-five per cent of new orthopaedic referrals are for back pain.
Only 20 per cent have a firm diagnosis made.
Twenty per cent of patients admitted to hospital undergo surgical intervention.

Eighty per cent of repeat back surgery leads to 'failure'.
Eighty thousand patients are permanently disabled by back pain.

Annual cost	
	£ *million*
General medical services	25.7
Pharmaceutical services	38.9
Outpatient consultations	25.3
Hospital inpatients	66.2
Certified incapacity from back pain	1,018
Payment of benefits	193
Home medicines	33

Clinical presentation

Back problems present with pain in the low back, with or without radiation to the legs, but a carefully taken history is the most useful part of the examination.

History

Age

Sex

History of initial presentation

Referral of pain pattern

What makes the pain worse?

What makes the pain better?

Past history

Diagnosis

The basis of any pathological problem in medicine is to make a diagnosis first and then introduce treatment. One of the problems of diagnosis is that so little is known about specific causes of pain.

Four basic features of back pain need to be identified:

Mechanical back pain
Space-occupying spinal pathology
   infections
   tumours
Inflammatory back pain
Discogenic failure with nerve root pain.

History should include:

Age
Sex
Occupation
Initial presentation
History of trauma
Type of pain
   site; referral pattern; episodic or not?

What makes the pain worse?
What makes the pain better?

Movement
Bending and twisting
Sitting
Walking
Morning stiffness
Night pain.

Associated features

Weight loss
Abdominal pain
Genitourinary problems.

Past history

back pain
inflammatory disease
trauma.

Having built up a picture, then the history can be expanded along more specific lines.

Mechanical back pain

The spine's function is to provide axial strength to the trunk, and at the same time allow flexibility in all three planes, to conduct and protect the spinal cord and nerve roots, and to act as a shock absorber. It is hardly surprising that the conflicting demands make back pain both complex and common.

Patterns of mechanical pain

Pain in the middle years of life
Pain is episodic and cyclic
Morning stiffness and pain
Pain increasing during the day
Pain on standing, walking and exercise
Pain on initiating movement
Pain on forward flexion and coming up from flexion

Pain on extreme lateral flexion and rotation
Poorly localized from L3 to the sacrum and referred to back, buttocks and thighs

Since the nerve supply to the spine includes all the muscles and ligaments around the spine, the facet joints, the outer layers of the discs and the periosteum, localization may prove difficult (Edgar and Park, 1974).

Disc degeneration is very common, usually occurring in the lowest space during the twenties and extending to the L4/5 space in the thirties. With the loss of disc height and mechanical integrity, more strain is placed on the small apophyseal joints, with consequent overlap. degeneration and onset of mechanical pain.

With ageing there is a fall in the water content of the interevertebral discs, disc nutrition becomes impaired, degenerative changes around the discs and facet joints increase, but symptoms usually improve. Degenerative changes throughout the spine do not presage symptoms, and this can be reassuring to patients.

Spondylolisthesis

Spondylolisthesis is the forward slip of one vertebra on the one below (Figure 10.1). Five per cent of the population go through life with a spondylolisthesis, and the incidence of back pain is the same as in the normal population. In adult life the presentation is more commonly due to concurrent disc degeneration than to mechanical failure. Spondylolisthesis is an important cause of back pain in adolescence (12 per cent) and must be specifically considered.

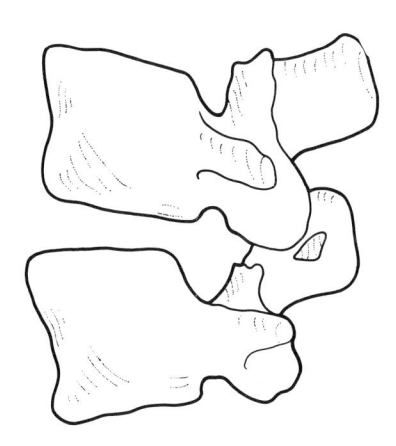

Figure 10.1 An isthmic spondylolisthesis associated with a fractured 'pars interarticularis'.

Soft tissues

The soft tissues, muscle and ligaments are very often implicated in minor structural pack pain. Unfortunately it is exceedingly difficult to identify the specific structure at fault, even with sophisticated techniques. Most of the conditions are self-limiting and not of serious import. On occasion, a soft tissue **trigger point** can be identified, and symptoms suppressed by the injection of a local anaesthetic.

Space-occupying pathology

Because of the prognosis and the effect of delay in treatment, these cases must be identified. About 10 per cent of patients attending the surgery have an underlying fear of serious pathology, particularly cancer, although inflammatory and metabolic conditions and neoplasms represent only 1–2 per cent of all cases of chronic back pain (Asherson, 1984). Luckily the presentation usually gives strong indications. (Jayson, 1984).

Age: the majority occur over the age of 55
Site: pain is well localized and may occur anywhere throughout the spine. Thoracic pain is of particular significance
Referral: root pain tends to be girdle in configuration
Episodic: space-occupying pain is continuous
Night pain: any patient with severe night pain must be considered to have a space-occupying lesion till proved otherwise
General malaise and
Past history of infection or trauma.

It must be borne in mind that nerve-root irritation can occur anywhere along the root and can be caused by a prolapsed disc, osteophytes or more peripherally by tumours.

The adolescent spine

Back pain in the adolescent is unusual and should in all cases be taken seriously. The commonest cause remains non-specific mechanical pain associated with growth but not specifically related to growth phenomena, such as Schmorl's nodes, or anterior wedge collapse in Scheuermann's disease.

Adolescent disc problems are uncommon, but presentation is very unusual; there is rarely significant pain, but often marked spasm is present, with a stiff spine frequently associated with a tilt.

Spondylolisthesis can be rapidly progressive in adolescent years and should be specifically excluded.

Spinal deformities, scoliosis and kyphosis are not usually associated with pain, but may be mentioned as a cry for help.

Who should be referred to hospital for further investigation?

Investigations:
x-ray lumbar spine
FBC & ESR

The majority of cases of mechanical pain settle spontaneously, but failure of conservative treatment or continued patient anxiety should suggest the advisability of a specialist opinion.

Spinal pathology

If this is suspected from the history, examination, or simple investigations, an urgent referral to outpatients is indicated.

Inflammatory pain

In most instances a specialist opinion is indicated in order to confirm the diagnosis. Thereafter treatment is based on anti-inflammatory drugs and physiotherapy.

Who should not be referred

Back pain is often a cry for help and not the primary problem. It is self-evident that such a patient should be identified where possible, and there is nobody better qualified than the patient's own doctor.

The most difficult group to identify and treat are the hysterics. Considerable research, mainly in the United States, has been made into the use of self-analysis questionnaires. The effectiveness of these is doubtful, and an observant and experienced practitioner is probably more reliable.

Since back pain is so difficult to quantify and assess, it becomes a favourite form of protest which is often unconscious. The protest may be against unhappiness at work – dissatisfaction either with the job itself or with the working conditions – or it may be against loneliness or unhappiness at home.

Medicolegal back pain is equally common, following injuries at work or road accidents and assaults. A solicitor's letter or DHSS form usually follows. It is very difficult to effect a cure before the case is settled.

Anybody who has been out of work for longer than a year **loses the work-ethic** and again produces problems of rehabilitation.

Examination

Rather than presenting an exhaustive description of the examination of a patient with back pain, some specific items will be highlighted.

Look
Note any tilt or spasm.
It is often worth watching a patient walk and noting any reciprocal back-muscle contractions.
Localized kyphosis or scoliosis should be noted.

Feel
Run the finger gently along the spine, confirm deformity and note any step along the spinous processes.
Localized tenderness should be carefully related to underlying structures, i.e. to the spine, the interspinous ligament, or over a joint.
Referred tenderness to the region of the iliolumbar and sacroiliac joints is common and does not necessarily denote underlying pathology.
The tenderness in patients with infection or tumour is usually very well localized, sharp, and often at unusual levels. Percussion causes acute pain.

Move
Stiff segments can be masked by hip flexion. To avoid being misled, mark the spine at L1 and also at L5 and measure spinal movement with a tape measure (Figure 10.2). Stiff segments within this area can often be noted by lying the patient on his face and palpating the spine firmly (Macrae and Wright, 1969).

Examine the lower limbs
Note any abnormal neurology.

Examine generally
Remember the classic sites from which a primary tumour can spread to bone, i.e.
  breast
  thyroid
  kidney
  prostate
  lung.
Think of generalized conditions and look at other joints.

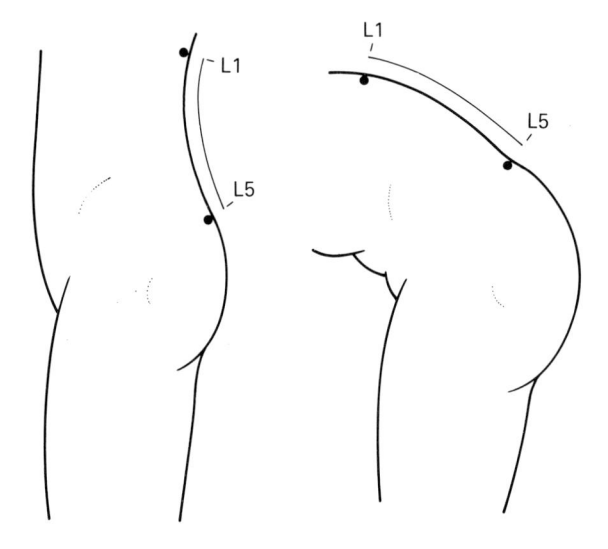

Figure 10.2 Measurement of forward flexion of the lumbar spine using a tape measure.

Feel the pulses
Vascular claudication can mimic symptoms of spinal stenosis (Verbiest, 1954) and abdominal aneurysms can produce back pain.

Investigations

Blood: FBC and ESR
Calcium phosphate, alkaline phosphatase
X-rays: lumbar spine.

At least 90 per cent of patients sent to hospital for investigation of back pain could be adequately screened by clinical examination and simple investigation. Clinical examination should reveal the presence of underlying pathology outside the spine, e.g. abdominal, pelvic, vascular, or metastatic disease.

The **ESR** is by far the most reliable blood test; it is very unlikely that serious spinal pathology can exist in the face of an ESR under 25 mm/hr and a normal plain x-ray.

Plain x-rays are very useful in excluding spinal pathology, but are unreliable in making a specific diagnosis.

A little under 50 per cent of x-rays of the spine are reported as abnormal in some way, many of the features commented upon are non-specific or irrelevant.

A focal lesion will only be detectable when 50 per cent of cancellous bone has been replaced. In patients with no suspicious features on history and clinical examination, only 1 in 2000 routine x-rays of the lumbar spine will demonstrate unexpected underlying pathology. X-rays are much more likely to demonstrate relevant abnormalities in the under-20 age group.

X-rays: What is relevant?

Abnormalities of bone texture suggesting metabolic, infective or malignant changes
Mechanical abnormalities: spondylolisthesis
Fractures: osteoporotic or traumatic
Deformities: kyphosis or scoliosis
Features specific to certain conditions, such as calcification in ankylosing spondylitis
Erosive changes from external pressure, for example neurofibromatosis or aneurysms.

Other abnormalities often commented upon, such as disc-space narrowing, degenerative changes or partial sacrolization, are often irrelevant to the immediate problem.

Hospital investigations

Full clinical history
Previous medical history
Systemic symptoms
Clinical examination
Plain x-rays
FBC and ESR

If these are negative, no pathology is likely.

At some stage in the investigation of any chronic back problem there is a need to make some form of **psychological assessment.** In simple terms, the hysterical patient usually does very badly whilst the depressed one may do very well, especially if the cause of depression is the back pain and this is alleviated. Either the help of a psychologist can be sought, or allowances put on a self-assessment questionnaire – a process not very popular in the United Kingdom. Considerable benefit may be gained in setting up a team approach to assess back problems, where contributions can be made from the various specialists – physician, radiologist, psychologist, physiotherapist, and occupational therapist.

Specific investigations (Figures 10.3 and 10.4)

Mechanical	*Spinal pathology*	*Root pain*
Oblique x-rays	Bone Scan	
Flexion/extension views of lumbar spine	Chest x-ray CAT scan Magnetic resonance imaging	Radiculogram
	Bone biochemistry	Venogram
Discogram	Plasma Proteins	Discogram
		EMG
	Rheumatoid and collagen screen	Root blocks
		CAT scan
	Widal and Brucella tests	
	Tuberculosis tests including EMU GCFT and VDRL	
	Needle bone biopsy ——— Histology ——— Bacteriology	

Treatment

Over 90 per cent of cases of back pain will settle within six weeks with simple, conservative treatment, rest, analgesia and reassurance (Waddell, 1982). It is because of this tendency that so many fringe practitioners flourish. Controlled trials of physiotherapy show a 30 per cent placebo effect (Shapiro, 1960). There seems to be no better treatment than quiet reassurance and a compassionate ear. The placebo response is not an indication of psychogenic pain, but is a normal response. The more dramatic the treatment, the greater the placebo effect.

Mechanical back pain

It is usually impossible to reverse deranged mechanics. Facet joint pain appears to respond unfavourably to spinal fusion, usually because the problem is at more than one level. Therefore, treatment needs to be applied throughout the lower lumbar spine.

Soft-tissue abnormalities. These can be successfully treated by identifying the soft-tissue structure at fault and injecting local anaesthetic and hydrocortisone.

Facet joint abnormalities. Analgesics are used; occasionally a good response to non-steroidal anti-inflammatory drugs is obtained.

Supports. The aim of a support, which can be canvas, plaster or plastic, is to produce local rest. Unfortunately, this is poorly achieved without

Examination 107

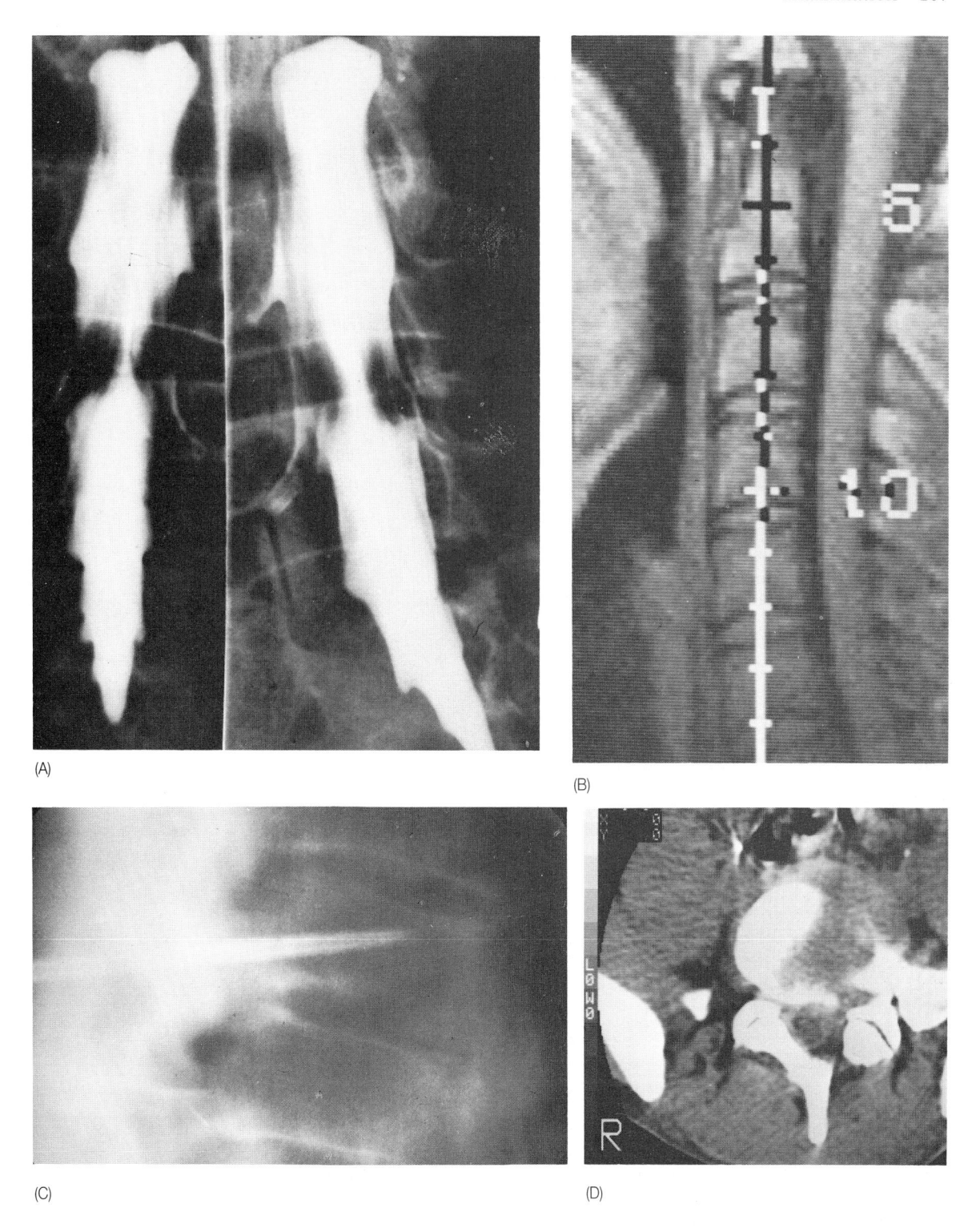

Figure 10.3 A. Radiculogram showing a central disc protrusion at L4/L5. B. Nuclear magnetic resonance scan of the neck showing the cervical spine and cord lying posteriorly. C. Needle biopsy. A needle has been inserted under x-ray control in the body of T9, which is the site of a secondary metastatic deposit. D. Computerized axial tomography scan showing a recurrent disc prolapse at L5/S1.

108 Low back pain

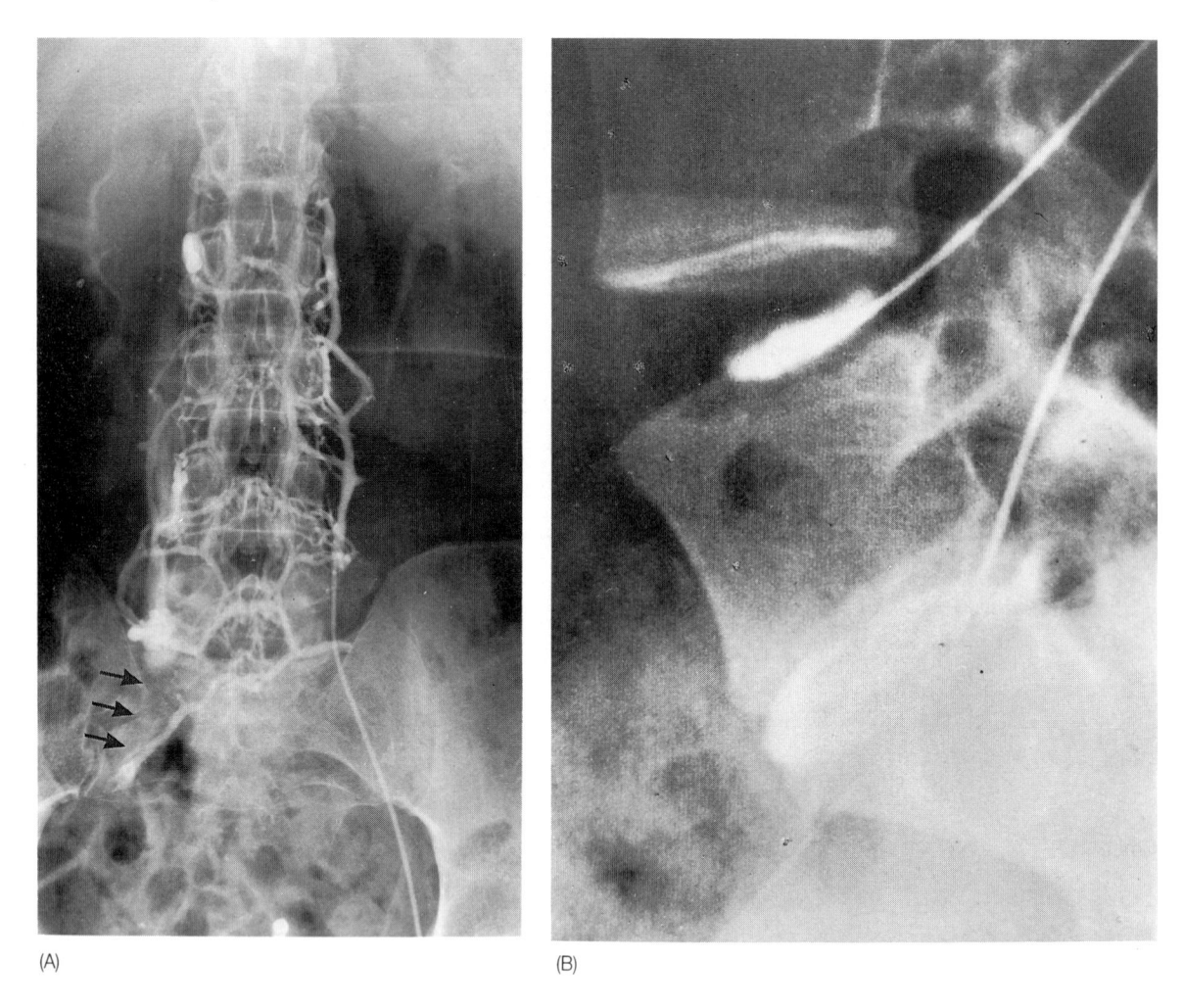

(A) (B)

Figure 10.4 A. Venogram demonstrating the pattern of veins in the lumbar region. The vein accompanying the left S1 root has not filled, indicating a disc prolapse at L5/S1. B. Discogram. Dye has been injected via two needles into the discs at L4/L5 and L5/S1. The L4/L5 disc is normal: the L5/S1 disc is ruptured, with dye leaking posteriorly.

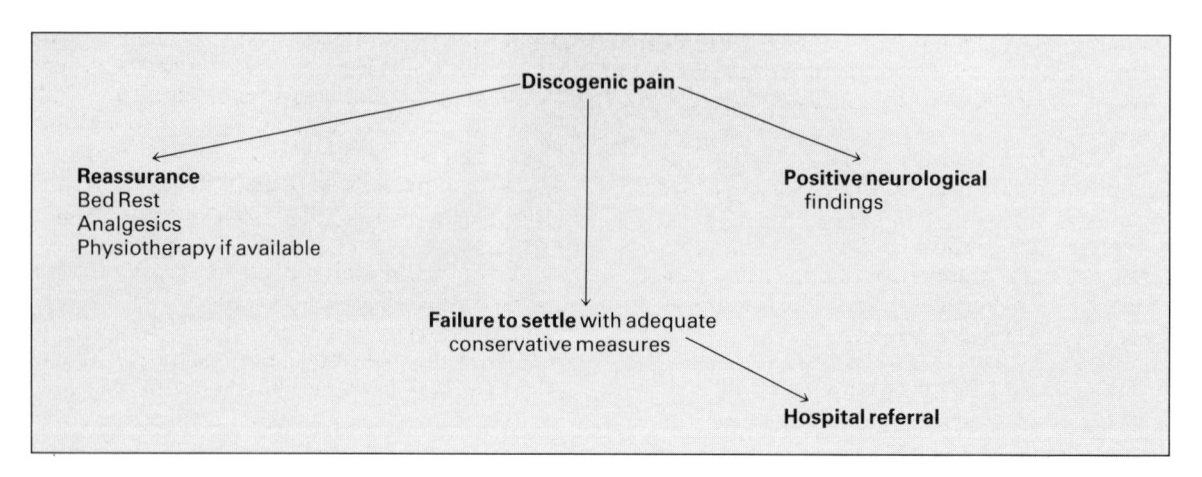

Discogenic pain

Reassurance
Bed Rest
Analgesics
Physiotherapy if available

Positive neurological findings

Failure to settle with adequate conservative measures

Hospital referral

Discogenic pain

immobilizing the joint below, e.g. a hip joint, and supports are of little value on a short-term basis. Any long-term treatment is at the cost of muscle tone, in both the abdomen and the back.

Physiotherapy. This is usually manipulative.

Injections. Any injections should be directed by x-ray control into the posterior joint. Initially a combination of steroid and local anaesthetic is used, but effects can be made more permanent with either cryoprobes or radio-waves.

Rhizotomy. This is the surgical division of posterior rami, but there is little to recommend it now that more sophisticated techniques are available.

Local injections of sclerosants can be made into ligaments to produce local 'tightening'. They are probably of little value.

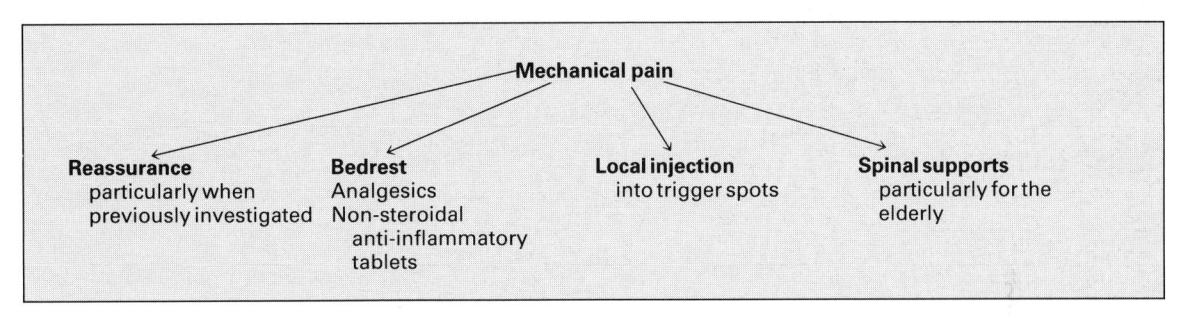

```
                          Mechanical pain
         ┌──────────┬──────────┴──────────┬──────────┐
    Reassurance    Bedrest          Local injection   Spinal supports
  particularly when Analgesics      into trigger spots particularly for the
  previously investigated Non-steroidal                 elderly
                    anti-inflammatory
                    tablets
```

Mechanical pain

Spinal pathology

Once the spinal pathology has been definitely identified, treatment can be specifically directed, and may involve drugs, radiotherapy or surgery.

Treatment of root pain

Bed rest and analgesia.

Physiotherapy. This is usually traction or manipulation. It should be remembered that (a) it is impossible to 'reduce' a disc prolapse, but (b) it may be possible to relieve root pressure or irritation.

Epidural injection. The aim is to 'wash' the root of the prolapsed disc and thus reduce nerve-root irritation.

Fenestration. The results of surgery are dependent on careful patient selection. A good result can be expected if three of the four following diagnostic criteria are present:

  Predominant root or leg pain
  Root irritation signs
  Root compression signs
  Positive contrast radiology, fitting in with the clinical picture.

Chymopapain. Injection of papain into the disc after discography disorganizes the ground substance and reduces water content. The indications and results are as for surgical excision. Chymopapain is particularly indicated for small, lateral disc prolapse, but is specifically *contraindicated* in cases of sequestrated discs.

Laminectomy and decompression. The more generalized narrowing of the canal seen in spinal stenosis is decompressed surgically by laminectomy. Lateral root entrapment requires surgical decompression by foraminotomy.

Spinal fusion alone is only indicated in progressive or proven painful spondylolisthesis and in the stabilization of spinal deformity.

Alternative medicine

We should not ignore alternative forms of medicine, but at the same time they need to be reviewed in the context of properly controlled trials in order to exclude the effect of natural history and the placebo. With back pain so common, and the primary and hospital services under such pressure, it is inevitable that patients will seek help outside the medical profession.

Herbalists, acupuncturists, chiropractors, osteopaths and faith healers all have their protagonists. Many of the techniques used, in particular by the osteopath, are those of the physiotherapist. The risks to the patient are of delay in the diagnosis of serious spinal pathology, and the occasional disaster of manipulation of a large central disc.

Having excluded these possibilities, there is an undoubted place for the practitioner of alternative medicine, and much good is done for sufferers with back pain.

Pain clinics

When all else has failed and the patient has been thoroughly investigated, an attempt can be made to block the pain pathways. Very little is understood about pain pathways and about the central mechanisms for the appreciation of pain.

The treatment given in pain clinics is dependent on interrupting these pathways by the use of (a) nerve block, (b) transcutaneous nerve stimulation and (c) acupuncture.

The occasional dramatic success makes this form of treatment well worth considering.

Rehabilitation and training

If all else fails, the patient must accept the continuation of symptoms and try to rebuild his or her life. Intensive rehabilitation can give hope and re-establish confidence. The only effective way to do this is on an inpatient basis, with care extending over a period of weeks. Unfortunately, facilities are limited, and demands outstrip them.

Retraining

Retraining requires careful assessment and a thoughtful and original retraining programme. Unfortunately again, facilities are limited, and too many patients have lost their pride and the 'work-ethic' before a proper programme can be instituted.

Comment

Low back pain is a common problem. The causes are multifactorial and the treatments involve too many unknown factors. The approach should be based on careful clinical assessment and supported by logical investigations. As each new clinical syndrome is described it becomes more important to dispel the doubt and confusion which usually obscure the approach to low back pain.

References
Asherson, R. (1984). *Mims Magazine,* June edition.
Auchinloss (1983). *The Painful Back.* Publishing Foundation, Oxford.
Back Pain (1985). London: Office of Health Economics.
Edgar, M.A. and Park, W.M. (1974). *J. Bone and Joint Surg.* **56**B, 658.
Jayson, M.I.V. (1984). *Brit. Med. J.* **1,** 740–741.
Macrae, I.F. and Wright, V. (1969). *Ann. Rheumat. Dis.* **28,** 584.
Shapiro, A.K. (1960). *Behavioral Science,* **5,** 109.
Veribiest, H. (1954). *J. Bone and Joint Surg.* 36B, 230.
Waddell, G. (1982). *Brit. J. Hosp. Med.* **28,** 3, 187–219.

11 Varicose Veins and Their Effects

Mark M. Orr and Brian R. McAvoy

Introduction

Varicose veins are tortuous, dilated and lengthened superficial veins (Figure 11.1). They are commonest in the legs but can also occur in the abdominal wall, oesophagus, anal canal (haemorrhoids) and pampiniform plexus (varicocele). They are alleged to be the price that man pays for the privilege of an upright posture, and were first described in the papyrus of Ebers over three-and-a-half thousand years ago.

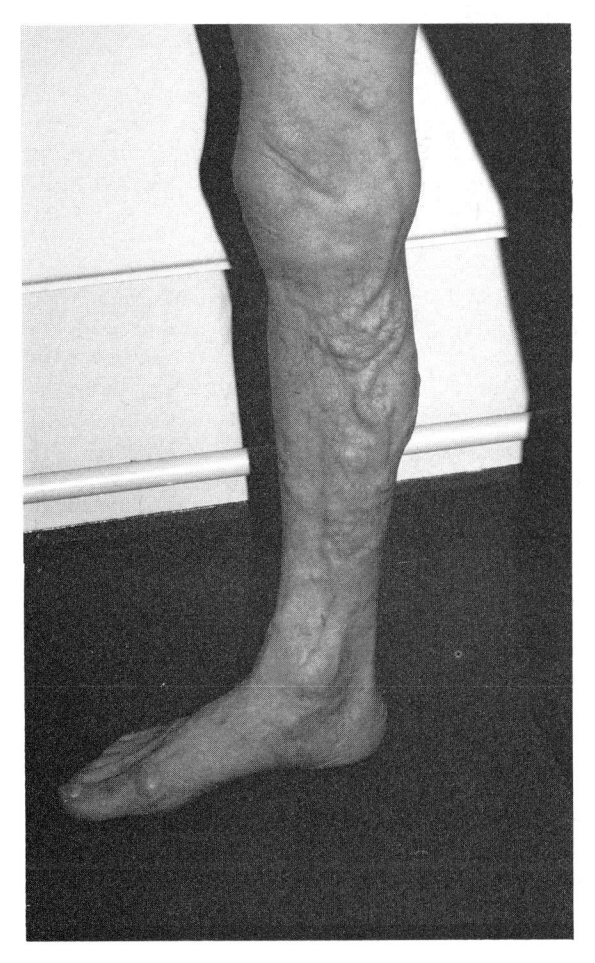

Figure 11.1 Typical varicose veins.

Anatomy

The leg has both superficial and deep systems of veins. The superficial veins – the long and short saphenous veins and their tributaries – lie outside the deep fascia, and drain into the deep veins – the femoral and popliteal veins (Figure 11.2). The termination of the long saphenous vein is fairly constant. That of the short saphenous vein is quite variable, commonly being higher than the knee, occasionally lower. The popliteal vein has two to three valves and the femoral vein two, in contrast to the short and long saphenous veins which have up to twelve and twenty valves respectively. It is these superficial veins in which varicosities develop.

The superficial and deep systems are connected by the perforator or communicating veins which include the two saphenous veins (Figure 11.2). There are multiple perforators in the thigh and calf, although only a few commonly become incompetent. Blood is thus drained from the low pressure superficial system to the higher pressure deep system. The so-called muscle pump, consisting of active calf muscles within a rigid fascial envelope, forces blood upwards towards the heart by a milking action, directed by the valves, and then sucks blood from the superficial into the deep veins while the muscles are relaxed.

The valves in the perforating veins prevent backflow of blood, but if they become incompetent the back pressure is transmitted to the superficial veins, damaging more distal valves and in time leading to the development of varicosities (Figure 11.3). The long and short saphenous veins have relatively thick muscular walls and they withstand raised hydrostatic pressure much better than their tributaries. The thick walls make stripping of the main vein possible. (The same quality allows the use of a supposedly varicose long saphenous vein in arterial bypass surgery.)

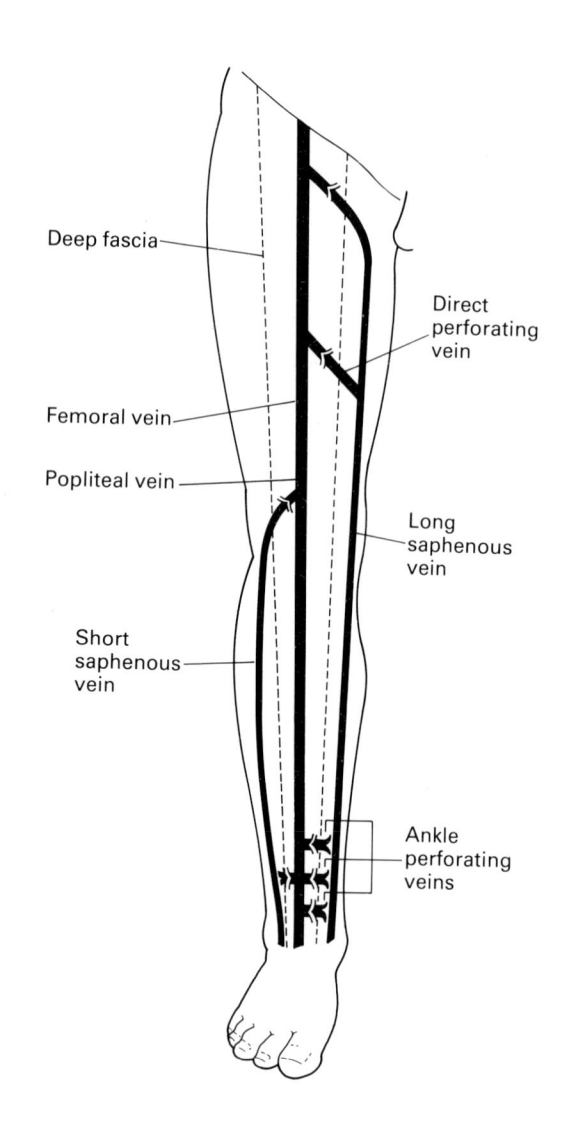

Figure 11.2 Normal anatomy of venous system of the leg.

Aetiology

Varicose veins may be primary or secondary.

Primary varicose veins

These are idiopathic, i.e. the cause is not known. Only rarely are the valve cusps absent or obviously abnormal. There is presumably a congenital defect in the vein wall, and this may be a deficiency of collagen. In addition, certain factors are thought to predispose to the development of varicosities (Table 11.1).

Family history – in about 70 per cent of cases.
Occupation – commoner in jobs which involve prolonged standing, particularly in warm surroundings.

Aetiology 113

Table 11.1 Factors predisposing to varicose veins

Family history
Occupation
Age
Sex
Pregnancy
Diet
Obesity.

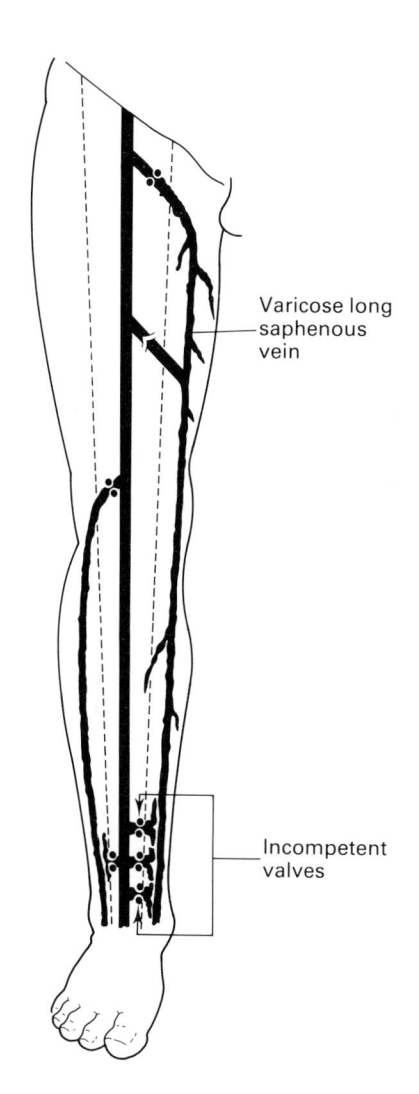

Figure 11.3 Development of varicose veins.

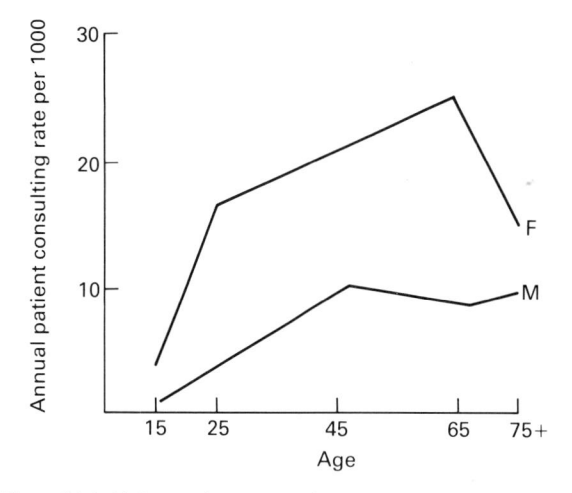

Figure 11.4 Varicose veins; age prevalence.

Age – commoner with increasing age (Figure 11.4).
Sex – commoner in women.
Pregnancy.
Diet – the typical low-fibre Western diet predisposes to constipation and straining at stool, raising intra-abdominal pressure; varicose veins are very rare in the Third World.
Obesity – this is often associated with varicose veins but the exact mechanism is uncertain.

Secondary varicose veins

These are associated with a known cause (Table 11.2). The mechanism may be dilatation of the vein resulting from prolonged back pressure, so that the valve cusps do not meet, or distortion of the valve cusps by thrombosis. Causes include:

Obstructed venous return
Pregnancy (the commonest cause)
Pelvic tumours – fibroids, ovarian carcinoma, etc.
Ascites
Thrombosis of the iliac veins or inferior vena cava
Retroperitoneal fibrosis
Deep vein thrombosis, resulting in damage to valves of deep veins and perforators. This may lead to the postphlebitic state
Arteriovenous fistulae – these raise venous pressure
Rare congenital anomalies such as the Klippel-Trenaunay syndrome.

Table 11.2 Causes of secondary varicose veins

Obstructed venous return
  pregnancy
  abdominal tumours
Deep vein thrombosis
  iliofemoral
  calf veins
Congenital anomalies and arteriovenous fistulae.

Varices associated with the last two causes may be in unusual sites such as the posterior aspect of the thigh, or very diffuse. The varices developing in pregnancy are not purely obstructive. The cause is partly hormonal, with a decrease in smooth muscle tone. Some *primary* varicose veins become much worse with pregnancy; other varices appear for the first time during pregnancy and are therefore secondary. This causes some confusion and difficulty in assessing the incidence of the two types.

Prevalence

It is estimated that 10 to 20 per cent of the population are affected by varicose veins, but some studies have suggested an even higher prevalence. For example, varicose veins were discovered in 62 per cent of Swiss chemical workers aged 20 to 65, including 22 per cent reported as having signs of chronic venous insufficiency (Da Silva et al., 1974). They are only slightly commoner in women, but consulting rates are three times higher for women than men and hospital admission rates are twice as high.

A general practitioner with an average list size of 2500 patients can expect to see about 30 patients per year presenting with varicose veins (RCGP, OPCS, 1974), but only a small proportion of these will be referred on to hospital.

A district general hospital serving a population of 250 000 will admit about 150 patients per year for varicose vein operations, and a general surgeon will perform three times as many hernia repairs and twice as many haemorrhoid procedures as varicose vein operations.

Each year in England and Wales nearly 32 000 operations are performed on veins, and every day 6560 hospital beds are occupied by patients having such surgery. The mean waiting time for surgery is nearly 33 weeks, and the mean duration of hospital stay is just over one week (DHSS, OPCS, 1984).

Classification

Varicose veins can be classified into four main groups (Table 11.3): those arising from incompetence of

> Long saphenous (commonest)
> Short saphenous (less common)
> Ankle perforators (very uncommon)
> Any combination – may present in one or both legs.

Table 11.3 Classification of varicose veins

Anatomical
  Long saphenous
  Short saphenous
  Ankle perforators
  Any combination of the above

Depth
  Intradermal – web
  Subdermal – reticular veins
  Subcutaneous – stem veins.

Although varicose veins are often associated with pregnancy, there are specific types of varicosities which occur *only* in pregnancy. These affect the vulval and pudendal veins and may become very large, but often regress and sometimes completely disappear after pregnancy.

Secondary varicose veins are classified according to the underlying cause (See page 113).

Recurrent varicose veins are those which develop after treatment.

Varicose veins can also be classified according to depth (Table 11.3):
  Intradermal
    web veins, spider or naevoid in form
  Subdermal
    reticular veins – showers of fine cuticular venules
  Subcutaneous
    stem veins, generally of long or short saphenous distribution.

Complications (Table 11.4)

These are commonest with stem varicosities and rare with reticular or web veins. The majority of varicose veins, however, do not cause serious problems or complications.

Table 11.4 Complications

Superficial thrombophlebitis
Skin changes
    eczema
    trophic changes
    fat necrosis leading to induration
    ulceration
Bleeding
Calcification
Periostitis of tibia
Marjolin's ulcer.

Superficial thrombophlebitis

This is a common complication. It usually involves superficial varicosities, but can occasionally extend into the deep system of veins. High ligation of the long or short saphenous veins may be indicated when a thrombophlebitis is propagating towards the deep vein junctions. High ligation can prevent development of a deep vein thrombosis and possible embolic complications.

Most cases of superficial thrombophlebitis, however, can be managed conservatively with support bandaging (elastic rather than crepe), mobilization, and anti-inflammatory analgesics such as aspirin or non-steroidal agents, e.g. ibuprofen, indomethacin, or naproxen. The traditional glycerin and ichthyol dressings are still popular, soothing and effective.

Skin changes

These result from prolonged venous hypertension, and are usually gradually progressive unless the underlying defect is corrected.

Eczema (Figure 11.5). Dry, scaly, pigmented areas of skin develop in relation to varicosities in up to 15 per cent of cases, most commonly over the gaiter area (Figure 11.6). These early changes are often aggravated by injudicious application of proprietary or prescribed creams and lotions. Although intended to alleviate itching and irritation, many such preparations contain powerful skin sensitizers, e.g. wood alcohol, parabens, chlorocresol, ethylene diamine, or propylene glycol. Allergic reactions contribute to ulceration and delay healing; they can be caused by many agents (Table 11.5). Topical steroids can be useful for short-term control of acute eczema, but prolonged use of fluorinated steroids produces skin atrophy.

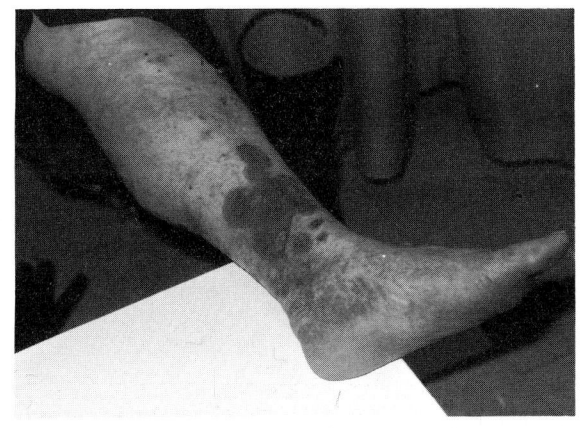

Figure 11.5 Varicose eczema.

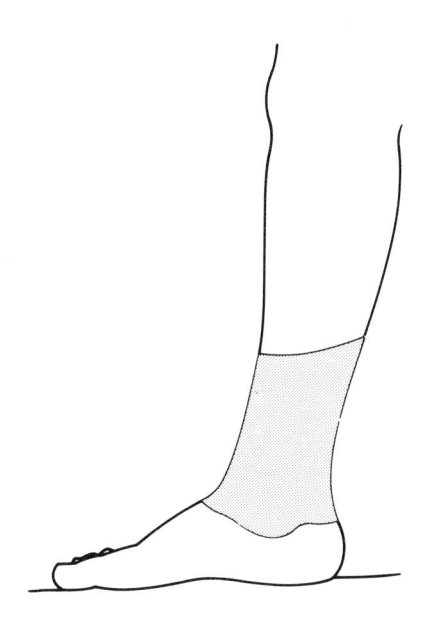

Figure 11.6 Area commonly affected by varicose eczema and ulceration.

Trophic changes. In 10 per cent of individuals with varicose veins chronic venous hypertension eventually produces increasing pigmentation, fibrotic thickening, induration, oedema, and atrophy of the skin. Recent work suggests that such changes develop as a result of perivascular fibrin cuffing of capillaries in the subcutaneous tissue, which interferes with normal tissue exchange of oxygen and nutrients and thus impairs healing (Browse and Burnand, 1982).

Fat necrosis. This eventually leads to 'woody' induration of the tissues.

Table 11.5 Leg ulcer allergens (Ryan, 1983a)

Ointment bases and preservatives
   Wool alcohols (lanolins)
   Parabens
   Propylene glycol
   Chlorocresol
   Ethylene diamine.

Antibacterial agents
   Sodium fusidate
   Gentamicin sulphate
   Neomycin
   Soframycin (framycetin and gramicidin)
   Vioform-Hydrocortisone (clioquinol and hydrocortisone)

Additives in bandages
   Ester gum resin
   Azo disperse yellow No. 3
   Colophony
   Mbt thiuram (rubber)

Self-medication
   Various '-caine' preparations (local anaesthetics)
   Antihistamine creams
   Dettol
   Germolene

Ulceration (Figure 11.7). The end point of such trophic changes is ulceration, affecting 3 per cent of those with varicose veins and often precipitated by trauma or infection. The terms 'varicose', 'gravitational' or 'stasis' ulcers are used, but the most appropriate term is 'venous ulceration'. Venous ulcers occur in the same area as venous eczema and are notoriously slow in healing. They may be very extensive and chronic. They are more common medially than laterally and are occasionally circumferential. Management is based on:

careful cleaning and dressing (using non-sensitizing preparations)
avoidance of infection; antibiotics are sometimes required
elastic compression bandaging; this is the most important single factor
mobilization
bed rest with elevation for the more resistant ulcers.

A variety of agents are available for cleaning ulcers (Table 11.6). The most useful is Eusol. Occlusive bandaging can be particularly helpful where the patient tends to scratch or remove dressings. Various medicated bandages are available (Table 11.7); these can be left on for up to one week, additional support being provided by pressure bandages (Table 11.8)

Table 11.6 Agents for cleaning ulcers (based on Ryan, 1983b)

Eusol (half- then quarter-strength)
Savlon
Normal saline
Dakin's solution
Silver nitrate solution
Potassium permanganate 0.1 per cent in water
Benzoyl peroxide 20 per cent solution
Aluminium acetate lotion
Hioxyl
Aserbine
Malatex
Debrisan

Table 11.7 Medicated bandages

Calaband
Coltapaste
Ichthopaste
Icthaband
Quinaband
Tarband
Zincaband

Table 11.8 Pressure bandages

Elastocrepe
Elastoplast
Flexoplast
Lestreflex
Poroplast
Varico leg bandage
Varihesive
Viscopaste PB7
NB *Elastocrepe* and *Tubigrip* is a good combination.

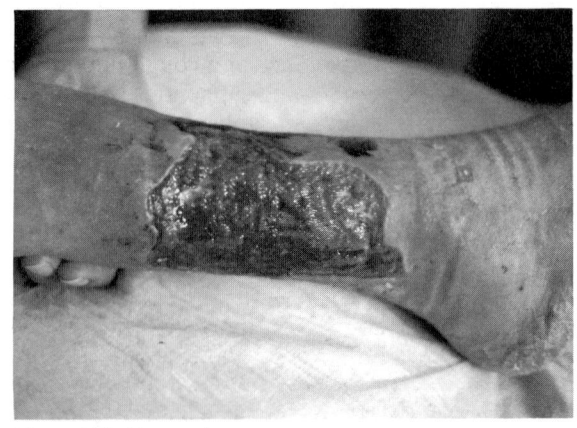

Figure 11.7 Venous ulcer.

> Firm, elastic compression is the single most important factor in the healing of venous ulcers

If *ambulant* treatment along these lines fails to promote healing, inpatient care may be required (see below).

Bleeding
This can be either spontaneous or traumatic, and occasionally can result in considerable blood loss. Immediate treatment involves elevation of the leg and application of pressure by means of a compression bandage.

Calcification
This is a very rare development in long-standing varicose veins.

Periostitis
Chronic venous ulceration over many years may result in periostitis of the underlying tibia.

Marjolin's ulcer
Squamous carcinoma may develop in very long-standing ulcers.

Clinical features

Patients with varicose veins present to their general practitioners with symptoms arising directly from the veins or their complications, or for cosmetic reasons.

History

Important points to cover in the history are:

   Reason for consultation; the common symptoms are listed in Table 11.9. Symptoms are

Table 11.9 Common symptoms of varicose veins

Aching or heaviness in legs – this can be general or localized
Mild ankle swelling
Itching over varices
Restlessness and night cramps in legs and feet
Symptoms due to thrombophlebitis – localized pain, tenderness, swelling and redness
Symptoms due to skin changes – itch and ulceration
Concern about cosmetic appearances – prominent varicosities, skin discoloration, unsightly flare varices
Bleeding.

   aggravated by prolonged sitting or standing (worse at the end of the day), and high temperatures, and are particularly bad premenstrually
   Duration and progression of symptoms
   Previous surgical or injection treatment
   Family history
   Obstetric history
   Occupation
   Relevant past medical history, e.g. trauma, deep vein thrombosis, or diabetes.

Examination

The patient should be examined both standing and lying flat; compare back and front of both legs. Gentle exercise such as walking around the room or repeated heel raising helps to reveal distension of the veins.

General assessment
General appearance. Is the patient fit or unfit looking? What is the weight?
Note the type, distribution and size of the varicosities with the patient standing (a diagram can be helpful). It is often clear which system is involved from the distribution of the varices.
Note presence of 'ankle flare', dilated venules below the malleoli.
Are there any skin changes, pigmentation, eczema, fat necrosis, oedema, or ulceration?
Is there evidence of previous surgery or thrombophlebitis – linear pigmentation?
Cough test. The presence of a cough impulse or even thrill over the long saphenous opening in the groin suggests saphenofemoral valve incompetence. A saphena varix may be palpable. An incompetent *short* saphenous does not produce a cough impulse.
Tourniquet tests. Locate the site of retrograde flow from the deep to the superficial systems. They are more sensitive than the cough test. In the Trendelenburg test, the patient lies down, elevates the leg to drain the superficial veins, and a tourniquet is tied tightly around the upper thigh below the groin. Localized digital pressure is a more precise alternative to a tourniquet. The

patient then stands. If the varicosities are due solely to saphenofemoral valve incompetence, they will fill only when the pressure is released. Early filling of the varicosities with the tourniquet still applied indicates incompetence at other sites. If this test is negative, the tourniquet test may be repeated using a single tourniquet (or digital pressure) in the lower thigh, to assess the perforator passing into Hunter's canal, and in the upper calf to assess the short saphenous vein. If the distal varices fill despite an upper calf tourniquet, there is likely to be an incompetent perforating vein in the calf.

Multiple tourniquet tests. A double tourniquet test may be used for routine assessment of both main saphenous systems, and a triple tourniquet test, although more complicated, is helpful in the assessment of very extensive or recurrent varices. The tourniquets are removed in turn, starting distally after half a minute's standing, and any filling of veins observed. The position of the tourniquets can be varied to localize the site of any incompetent perforator.

When these tests are clearly positive or clearly negative, firm conclusions can be drawn, but sometimes there is slow, unconvincing filling. It is vital, particularly in complicated cases, to empty the varicosities thoroughly by high elevation and manual expression before applying the tourniquet.

Perthes' test. This can be used to confirm the presence of incompetent perforators in the lower leg and to obtain information on deep vein patency. In the standing position a tourniquet is applied below the knee, firmly enough to occlude the superficial veins, and the patient is asked to mark time on the spot. If the perforators are competent, superficial veins should empty as blood is sucked into the deep compartment and pumped upwards. If the varices become more prominent, there is perforator incompetence. If in addition the leg becomes engorged and congested, the deep veins are probably occluded. In general, clinical localization of incompetent perforators is difficult and inaccurate. Some 'blow-outs' may be very obvious. Careful palpation of the lower leg in the recumbent position may suggest defects in the fascia transmitting such perforators, but this is only about 50 per cent accurate (Beesley and Fegan, 1970).

Percussion. Tapping one end of a column of blood while palpating the other with two fingers can help to determine whether a group of varicosities is in direct communication with the long or short saphenous systems.

> The accurate assessment of varicose veins is all important in the selection of treatment for sclerotherapy or surgery

More extensive examination

This is indicated if underlying disease is suspected.

   Abdomen for masses or ascites
   Rectal examination for masses or pelvic tumours
   Peripheral arterial pulses if ischaemic changes are noted
   Neurological examination of legs if there are trophic changes
   Auscultation. A bruit may be heard if there is an underlying arteriovenous fistula.

In hospital a more general examination to ascertain fitness for anaesthesia would be undertaken prior to surgical treatment.

Investigation

Most individuals with varicose veins require no investigation. When secondary or recurrent varicose veins are suspected further investigation may include:

   Venography (ascending phlebography). This is useful for demonstrating obstructed veins, collaterals and incompetent perforators
   Varicography, for tracing recurrences
   Ultrasound, for demonstrating reflux into superficial veins
   Volume and pressure studies ⎫
   Thermography   ⎬ rarely performed
   Isotope and impedance   ⎪ clinically
      phlebography   ⎭

Patients requiring surgery may well have a preoperative haemoglobin check; older patients may also require a chest x-ray, ECG, and urea and electrolytes check.

Assessment and decisions

The key questions for general practitioners are:

Who needs treatment?
What treatment is most appropriate?
Who needs referral to hospital?

Most patients presenting in general practice with varicose veins can be managed without referral to hospital. Referral is indicated under the following circumstances:

Symptoms become intolerable to the patient (including cosmetic appearance)
Recurrent superficial thrombophlebitis
Progressive chronic venous insufficiency (prophylaxis of ulceration)
Uncontrolled ulceration, or for definitive treatment following ulceration
After rupture and bleeding from a varicosity.

Women should preferably defer definitive treatment until they have completed childbearing. Obese patients should be encouraged to lose weight before referral.

Management

In practice the mainstay of treatment is external compression. More active treatment involves:

injection sclerotherapy
surgery (ligation and stripping).

Some patients with early varicosities may need no treatment apart from an *explanation and reassurance* that they are unlikely to develop any serious problems or complications. General advice may also be needed about increasing dietary roughage, reducing weight, remaining active, avoiding prolonged sitting or standing in one position, and elevating the legs at rest whenever possible.

External compression

This is best provided by wearing support hose (full-length standard elastic yarn). These must be put on before getting out of bed in the morning and kept on all day, either by themselves or under normal stockings or tights. Support stockings, but not tights, are prescribable under the NHS. They provide good symptomatic relief and may well slow down the progression of varicosities. In practice they are often poorly tolerated, particularly in warm weather.

External compression is indicated:

in minor but symptomatic varicose veins
in the elderly or infirm
in pregnancy
in venous ulceration
in patients who decline sclerotherapy or surgery
with secondary varicose veins due to deep vein valve damage
as a therapeutic trial to determine the source of atypical leg pain
in the postoperative period, or following injection.

Injection sclerotherapy

This can be performed as an outpatient procedure or in the general practitioner's surgery, and is appropriate for:

Diffuse, low pressure varicosities with no saphenous incompetence
Mild varicosities of the lower leg
Symptomatic varices as an alternative to surgery
Residual or recurrent veins after surgical treatment. Large venous telangiectases (occasionally warranted).

A sclerosing solution, e.g. sodium tetradecyl sulphate (STD) is injected into veins which have been marked out carefully and emptied by elevation. Firm compression with foam-rubber pads and *Elastocrepe* bandages is then applied and the area covered by a Tubigrip support. Several sites may be injected in one leg. The patient is encouraged to walk for about 20 minutes after the injection, and for similar periods several times per day for the next few weeks. Reassessment is advised after two weeks and further injections can be given as required. Compression is maintained for 4 to 6 weeks.

Relative contraindications to sclerotherapy

> Veins above mid-thigh
> Veins in the popliteal fossa
> Incompetent ankle perforators
> Veins around the medial malleolus or on the foot
> The elderly or inactive
> Fat legs
> Oral contraceptive treatment
> Peripheral vascular disease
> Post-thrombotic syndrome
> Extensive varicose eczema or ulceration
> Very fine cutaneous venules (for technical reasons).

Complications

> Painful thrombosis
> Skin blistering and ulceration
> Persisting brown discoloration along the line of the vein
> Hypersensitivity reactions
> Deep vein thrombosis and pulmonary embolism (rare)
> Gangrene (rare) (due to intra-arterial injection).

Patients seeking treatment for web and reticular veins should be warned of the possible cosmetic effect of injections, as the main reason for treatment is invariably cosmetic. Injections can be made intradermally using very small 'blebs' of sclerosant via a fine needle and using a magnifying loupe but this is very time consuming and rarely satisfactory.

Surgery

This is the more precise form of treatment and is indicated for patients with main-stem varices due to saphenous and/or major perforator incompetence. In practice these constitute the majority of those referred. Some operations can be performed as day cases but most require general anaesthesia. The main procedures are:

1. Trendelenburg procedure – flush ligation of the long saphenous vein at its entry into the femoral vein with ligation of all the local tributaries.
2. Short saphenous ligation – ligation of the short saphenous deep in the popliteal fossa but not necessarily flush with the popliteal vein.
3. Stripping of long or short saphenous vein – performed less often nowadays, as the main vein is generally not grossly dilated. The vein is stripped to the groin from the upper calf level rather than from the ankle, to avoid damage to the saphenous nerve. Stripping of the short saphenous is rarely undertaken.
4. Multiple ligations and avulsions of varices, to remove the actual veins of which the patient is most aware. Otherwise they persist and may become symptomatic later.
5. Ligation of perforators – most commonly those of the lower thigh and lower calf (i.e. ankle perforators), medial or lateral. The approach may be subcutaneous or subfascial (Dodd and Cockett, 1976).
6. Combinations of the above, on one or both legs.

Ligation of an incompetent saphenous vein as a day case may be combined with injection sclerotherapy to the related varices, with early ambulation, or residual varices may be injected in outpatients later. *Whichever procedure is used,* the veins must be fully marked out preoperatively, preferably by the surgeon who will perform the operation, to ensure that *full clearance of the veins* will be achieved. The *thoroughness* of the procedure is the most important aspect of treatment if it is to be successful. Many patients have varices which are suitable for either sclerotherapy or surgery, and the choice of treatment will depend on the preference of the surgeon or patient, the length of the waiting list, and the availability of a suitable sclerotherapy clinic.

Following operative procedures, firm crepe bandaging is applied and early mobilization encouraged on the first postoperative day, with additional support – blue-line or red-line bandages. In the absence of a stripping procedure, there is less postoperative pain and the patient may be discharged home after 48 hours. Bandaging is continued for four to six weeks. At outpatient follow up at six weeks, any residual varices may be injected to complete the treatment. Postoperative complications are uncommon:

> Haematoma, particularly in groin wound
> Wound sepsis – rare, mild

Damage to cutaneous nerves, e.g. saphenous or sural nerves

Superficial thrombophlebitis in a 'neglected' vein

Deep vein thrombosis and pulmonary embolism – rare.

Secondary varicose veins need careful selection for surgical treatment. If the prominent varices are essentially collaterals following deep vein thrombosis, simple compression treatment is safest. If, however, the veins are very symptomatic and the deep veins are patent, surgery is appropriate and the veins are treated on their merits.

Refractory venous ulcers

Venous ulcers which do not improve with ambulant outpatient treatment may require inpatient care or surgery. Before this point is reached, the patient must be given adequate support in the form of elastic crepe or red-line bandages over a compression pad for a reasonable trial period. Dressings are *best kept simple* and *not repeated too frequently,* e.g. only twice a week or less often. The size of the ulcer can be measured to assess progress.

If the above regimen fails, inpatient bed-rest with high elevation of the legs will give the best chance of healing. Often this is necessary to obtain healing of ulcers prior to surgery. Vitamin C and antibiotics may be useful. If there is failure of healing under these conditions, an ischaemic factor may be present and sometimes lumbar sympathectomy or direct arterial surgery will be necessary to promote healing.

Split-skin grafting may be used to accelerate healing, but prolonged bed rest will still be required to ensure a satisfactory 'take'. Once the ulcer has healed, surgical treatment of the underlying veins may proceed. This will often involve subfascial ligation of ankle perforators.

Occasionally the post-phlebitic limb is so severely afflicted with intractable ulceration, fibrosis and equinus that amputation is required. This may also prove to be the most logical treatment in Marjolin's ulcer. Following the successful treatment of venous ulceration by any method, it is wise to continue with firm compression using an elastic bandage or stocking, partly for support and partly for protection of the delicate skin in the gaiter area. Overall, the prognosis for venous ulcers is much better if they are associated with gross saphenous varices rather than with the post-phlebitic syndrome.

> Bed rest with high elevation of legs will heal any purely venous ulcer. Maintaining healing is another matter!

Drugs

The place of drug treatment in the management of varicose veins has not been determined. If nocturnal cramps are troublesome, quinine sulphate may be used to control them. Claims are made for oxerutins (Paroven) in relieving the *symptoms* of varicose veins and it may be useful in the overall assessment of the problem. It has been suggested that the anabolic steroid stanozolol (Stromba) is valuable in healing intractable lipodermosclerosis; it reduces induration, inflammation, tenderness and pigmentation, but is not of proven benefit in ulceration (Burnand et al., 1980).

Results of treatment

Initial results of treatment are satisfactory, but five years after sclerotherapy or surgery, further treatment is needed in about 50 per cent and 25 per cent of patients respectively.

Long-term success depends on:

appropriate selection of patients for sclerotherapy or surgery
thoroughness of the treatment.

Patients with major saphenous incompetence who are treated by injection tend to get early recurrences. Otherwise, in enthusiastic hands, the results of sclerotherapy may be almost as good as surgery.

Primary long saphenous varices do not usually recur after effective surgical treatment because the deep veins and perforators are normal. However, varicose veins secondary to thrombosis are more liable to recur because treatment occludes further veins.

The patients who do get recurrences tend also to do less well after later forms of treatment.

Acknowledgements

We wish to thank Angela Chorley and Margaret Gold of Audiovisual Services, University of Leicester, for Figures 11.2, 11.3 and 11.6, and the General Practice Unit, University of Leicester for Figures 11.1, 11.5 and 11.7.

References

Beesley, W. H. and Fegan, W. G. (1970). An investigation into the localisation of incompetent perforating veins. *Brit. J. Surg.,* **57,** 30.

Browse, N. L. and Burnand, K. G. (1982). The cause of venous ulceration. *Lancet* **2,** 243–245.

Burnand, K. G., Clemenson, G., Morland, M., Jarrett, P. E. M. and Browse, N. L. (1980). Venous lipodermatosclerosis: treatment by fibrinolytic enhancement and elastic compression. *Brit. Med. J.* **280,** 7–11.

Da Silva, A., Widmer, L. K., Martin, H., Mall, Th., Glaus, L. and Schneider, M. (1974). Varicose veins and chronic venous insufficiency. *Vasa,* **3,** 118.

Department of Health and Social Security, Office of Population Censuses and Surveys (1984). *Hospital Inpatient Enquiry.* Series MB4 No. 20. London: HMSO.

Dodd, H. and Cockett, F. B. (1976). *The Pathology and Surgery of the Veins of the Lower Limb.* Edinburgh and London: Churchill Livingstone.

Royal College of General Practitioners, Office of Population Censuses and Surveys (1974). *Morbidity Statistics from General Practice: Second National Study 1970–71.* London: HMSO.

Ryan, T. J. (1983a). *The Management of Leg Ulcers,* p. 66. Oxford: Oxford University Press.

Ryan, T. J. (1983b). *The Management of Leg Ulcers,* p. 59. Oxford: Oxford University Press.

12 The Ischaemic Leg

Mark M. Orr and Brian R. McAvoy

Introduction

Ischaemia of the lower limb is a common clinical problem. It is usually a chronic condition, due to obliterative disease of the arteries to the leg, which produces typical symptoms and signs as a result of anoxia in the muscles and other tissues.

Atherosclerosis is the commonest cause but other conditions may be responsible particularly in acute ischaemia. The effects of arterial disease depend on the site affected and the speed of progression of the disease.

Aetiology

The terms **atherosclerosis** and **atheroma** are used synonymously for the common form of generalized **arterial disease**. It affects arteries at many sites and is responsible for high morbidity and mortality in the population.

Other causes of ischaemia of the legs:

   Diabetes mellitus tends to affect smaller distal arteries
   Buerger's disease (thromboangiitis obliterans) also affects smaller arteries
   Arterial embolism generally causes acute ischaemia
   Trauma also causes acute ischaemia
   Vasospastic disease – Raynaud's disease, scleroderma, etc.
   Frostbite, trench foot – cold and immersion injury
   Sepsis – cellulitis leading to areas of skin necrosis.

Atherosclerosis

Atherosclerosis has a predilection for certain sites in the body and in the leg. The coronary, carotid and cerebral arteries are commonly affected, a fact which must be borne in mind in the management of peripheral arterial disease. In the leg the primary occlusion site is the lower superficial femoral artery in 60 per cent of patients, and the aortoiliac segment in about 30 per cent (Figure 12.1). Multiple sites of disease (or multi-level disease) occur in about 7 per cent of cases. The pattern of arterial involvement is commonly symmetrical, although one leg tends to be more affected than the other.

Pathology

Three types of lesion are found within arterial walls (Figure 12.2):

1. Fatty streaks – These are the earliest 'lesions' (may be seen in one-year-old infants). They do not restrict blood flow.
2. Fibrous or pearly plaques. These encroach on the lumen, restricting flow. They contain yellow pultaceous material.
3. Complicated plaques. These are plaques showing one of the following: ulceration, calcification, thrombosis or haemorrhage.

124 The ischaemic leg

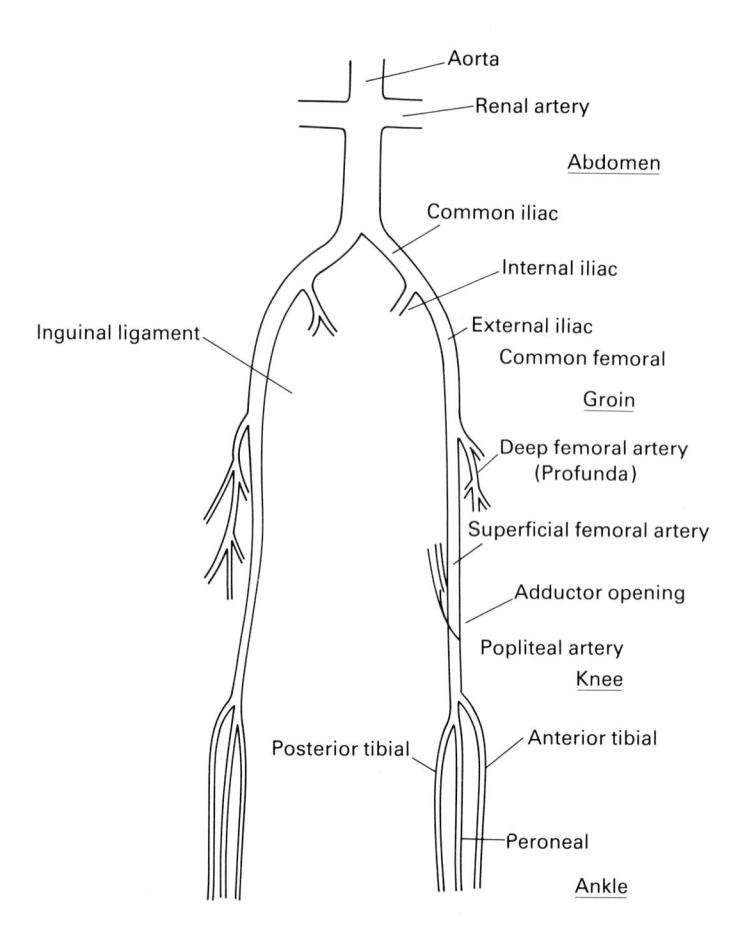

Figure 12.1 Arterial system of the legs.

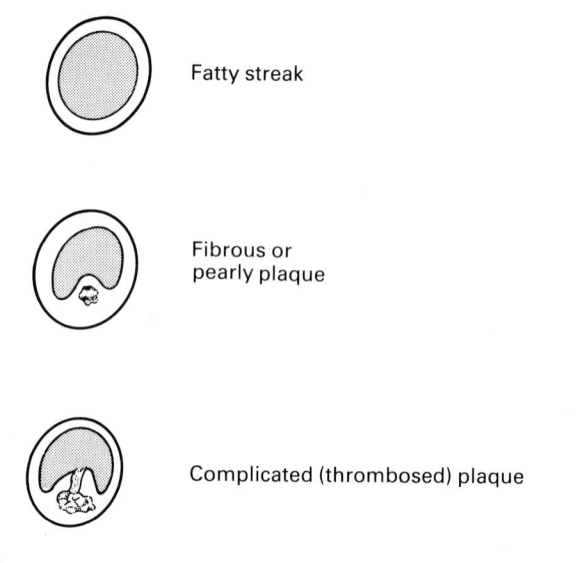

Figure 12.2 Types of atheroma lesions.

They are more common in the elderly.

The end result of this process is occlusion of an artery and/or the risk of embolism.

Risk factors which influence severity of atherosclerosis:

Male sex
Ageing
Hypertension
Diabetes mellitus
Cigarette smoking.

Collateral circulation

The degree of ischaemia brought about by arterial occlusion or stenosis, and therefore the symptoms, depend on the presence or absence of an effective collateral circulation. This is an accessory system or circuit of pre-existing side-branches of the main artery above and below the occlusion (Figure 12.3) brought into play by the local pressure gradient. The efficiency of the collateral circulation depends on:

Site and length of the occlusion or stenosed segment
Time course of the disease process.

The slower the encroachment of disease on the lumen, the more time available for collaterals to form; this means that eventual total occlusion may be well compensated. A sudden embolic block, however, finds the circulation unprepared, with more severe consequences.

The main collateral vessel of the leg is the deep femoral artery, or profunda, with its muscular branches. It is generally less prone to disease than the other arteries of the leg, and may take over so readily that ischaemic symptoms do not arise.

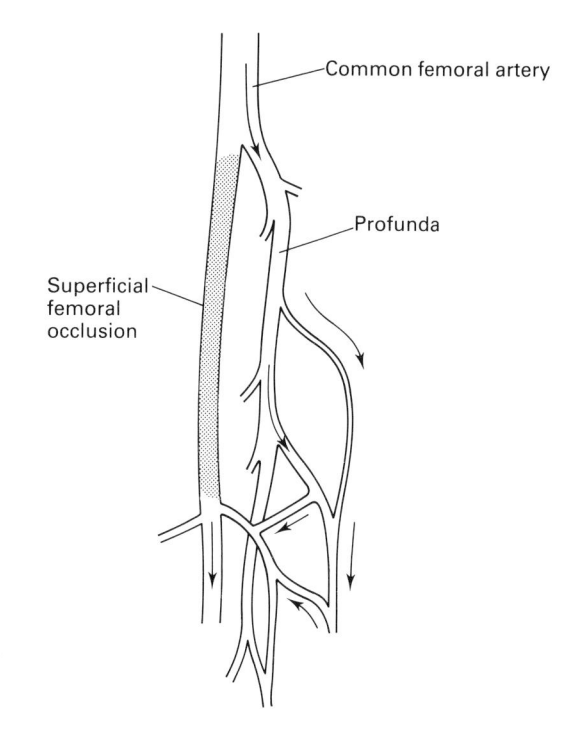

Figure 12.3 Collateral arterial circulation in the leg.

Clinical features

Symptoms

The average patient, an ageing male smoker, presents with **intermittent claudication**. This is a cramp-like pain in the muscles of the leg brought on by walking. One or both calves may be affected and the pain comes on after walking a certain distance. The patient then has to stop and stand still to rest the ischaemic calf muscles. Once the pain has gone the patient can resume walking and cover the same sort of distance again.

The distance walked before the pain starts is called the **claudication distance** and it varies somewhat with speed of walking, gradient and any weight being carried. The speed of recovery from claudication pain is directly related to the efficiency of the collateral circulation.

Claudication may affect the thigh muscles or the buttocks as well as or separately from the calf, according to the level of disease. Calf claudication indicates superficial femoral disease. Gluteal claudication is caused by aortoiliac disease. There may be associated impotence and wasting of the buttock muscles (Leriche's syndrome). Claudication is rare in the foot, and suggests peripheral small artery involvement as in Buerger's disease.

Numbness of the foot may be noticed as a result

of diversion of blood to the active muscle, i.e. **'muscle steal'**.

About 10 per cent of patients present with **ischaemic rest pain,** generally in addition to claudication. It is felt in the foot, typically in the forefoot or toes in bed overnight, and it may be relieved by exposure or dependency. The sufferer soon learns to hang the leg out of bed to gain relief or even to resort to sleeping in an armchair. Gravity improves perfusion but also encourages **oedema. Night cramps** in the foot or calf may be a problem.

Painful **ischaemic ulcers** may form on pressure points and patches of gangrene develop in one or more toes, although this may be a relatively painless process in the elderly or diabetics. Infection in a toe or callosity may follow inexpert attention to the nails, corns or bunions.

The symptoms of claudication and rest pain are characteristic in their sites, timing and relieving factors, so they are not easily confused with other conditions. (Table 12.1).

Table 12.1 Differences between intermittent claudication and ischaemic rest pain.

Symptom	Intermittent claudication	Ischaemic rest pain
Timing	With exercise, by day	At rest, by night
Tissue	Muscle	Skin
Site	Calf > thigh > buttock	Extremity – toes, heels
Posture	Walking	Recumbent
Relief	Standing still	Dependency, standing, cool surface
Type of pain	Cramping	Constant ache, intractable

If claudication seems atypical a careful history will often implicate the spine or hip joint as a source of pain. In spinal stenosis the pain may come on in the lower back purely on standing as well as walking, and may radiate down the legs as sciatica (claudication of cauda equina).

Patients may present with cold, painful feet and recurrent **chilblains** as manifestations of vasospastic disease. **Acute ischaemia** may occur spontaneously or following trauma and is usually dramatic with sudden onset of pain, coldness and numbness in one or both legs. However, presentation may be delayed with milder symptoms. The past history of claudicants often includes coronary disease with angina or past myocardial infarction, cardiac arrhythmia, hypertension or cerebrovascular disease. Most patients are, or have been, smokers. There may be a history of past ischaemic episodes in the legs.

Signs

Inspection of a **chronically ischaemic leg** may reveal very little abnormality, particularly if claudication is the only symptom. The following features may be noted:

Coldness of the foot (not specific to ischaemia)
Loss of normal hair
Shiny, atrophic skin
Oedema of foot and ankle
Muscle wasting in calf or thigh
Trophic changes in skin or nails
Poor perfusion (slow return of colour after blanching of skin)
Postural colour changes – elevation pallor and dependent rubor (i.e. 'sunset foot') (Figure 12.4)

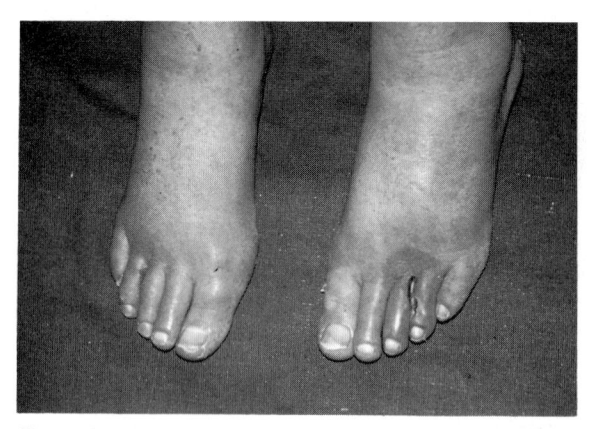

Figure 12.4 'Sunset foot'. Postural colour changes in ischaemic feet.

Venous 'guttering' on elevation
Dry, tender 'fissure ulcers' in skin – interdigital or on heel
Ulcers on toes or pressure points
Septic lesions – paronychia, pulp sepsis, bunion, etc.
Gangrene of one or more toes (Figures 12.5, 12.6)
Loss of pulses in leg – see below
Presence of bruits
Aneurysm: aorta > femoral > popliteal.

The pulses should be checked in all four limbs and recorded accurately with any aneurysms or bruits,

The ischaemic leg 127

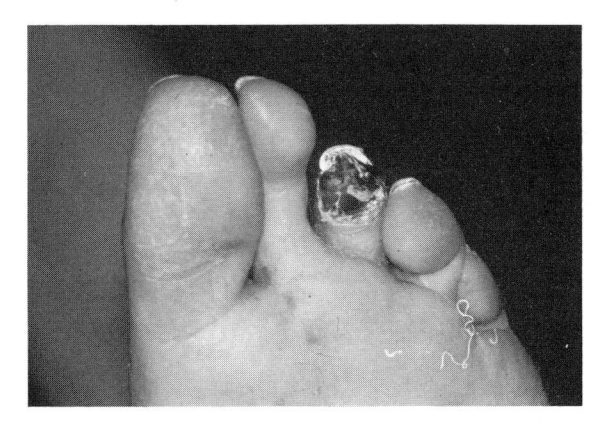

Figure 12.5 Gangrenous toes.

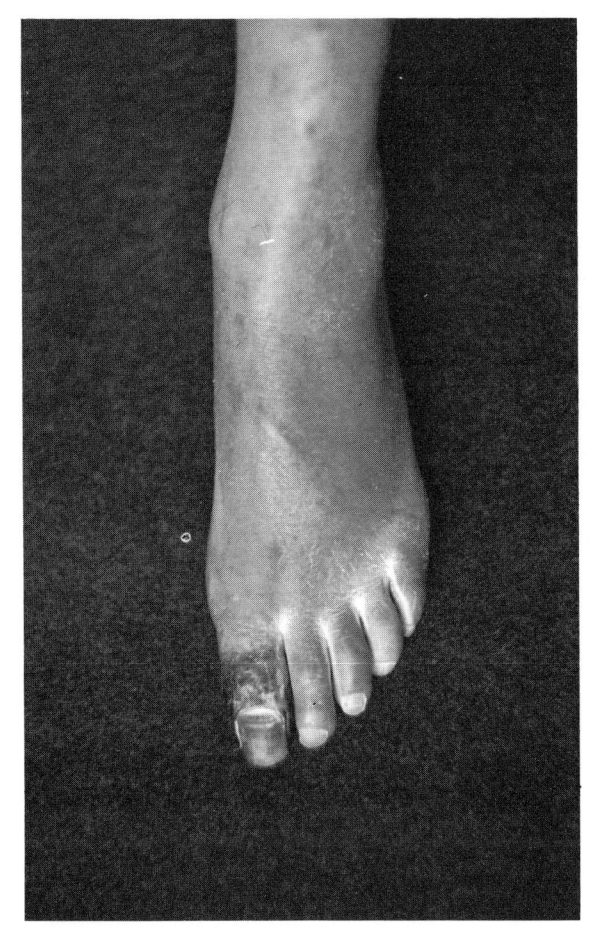

Figure 12.6 Gangrenous toes.

hands placed around the slightly flexed knee with the fingertips of one hand pressing the others **firmly** down into the fossa. Any difficult pulse is best timed against the patient's femoral or radial (to avoid confusion with one's own pulse).

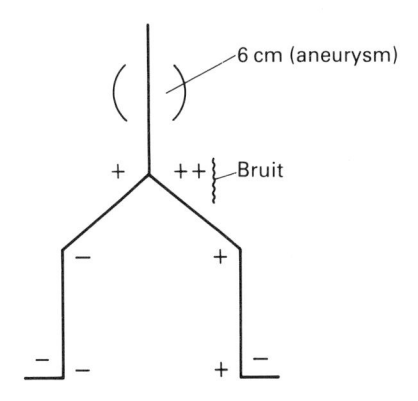

Figure 12.7 The ischaemic leg. Main arterial findings.

In **acute ischaemia** the clinical features are represented by:
Pain
Pallor
Paraesthesia or numbness
Paresis or weakness
Loss of pulses.

> The most sensitive signs of acute ischaemia are muscle dysfunction and sensory deficit

The cold skin of the distal part of the limb may show mottled discoloration. The neglected case may show bluish/purple discoloration of the extremity without blanching on pressure. This 'fixed staining' of the skin is a sign of irreversible ischaemia. The calf muscles may be tender, swollen, bunched, or of doughy feel, with equinus at the ankle.

Abdominal examination is important for the aortic 'pulse', aneurysm as a source of emboli, and to record the external iliac pulses.

Further clinical examination will often reveal evidence of cardiac disease or hypertension; atrial fibrillation is particularly common.

not omitting the carotids (Figure 12.7). The dorsalis pedis is often absent congenitally.

Difficulty is often experienced in palpating the popliteal pulse. This is best sought using both

Investigations

The following routine tests may be requested before or after referral to hospital:

Full blood count, glucose, urea and electrolytes, and fasting serum lipids
ECG
Chest x-ray and plain abdomen x-ray.

Specialized investigations

Doppler ultrasound assessment

This detects blood flow in the arteries. It gives useful information on the degree of ischaemia, particularly when diagnosis is in doubt (with atypical pain or possible spinal disease). Quantitative information is available from measurement of the Doppler systolic ankle pressure.

$$\text{Doppler pressure index} = \frac{\text{Ankle systolic pressure}}{\text{Brachial systolic pressure}}$$

The Doppler pressure index is measured at rest and, if necessary, after exercise. In normal subjects the ratio should be over 1.0 at rest, and remain unaltered with exercise. In ischaemia there is a fall with exercise from normal or low resting values; and the recovery time depends on the degree of ischaemia and the adequacy of the collateral circulation. The assessment is best done with exercise on a treadmill under standard conditions.

Uses of Doppler index

The initial assessment of ischaemia
To monitor the progress of the condition
To measure the response to arterial reconstruction
As a guide to amputation level.

Typical values in health and disease are shown in Table 12.2

Segmental pressure cuffs may be used in the leg to demonstrate **the site** of a pressure drop, e.g. a distal superficial arterial occlusion.

Arteriography

This remains the most useful method of investigation and it is essential before arterial reconstruction is undertaken. It must show the state of the arterial system well above and below the occlusion, and this generally entails aortography with views down to ankle level.

Table 12.2 Typical values for Doppler index in health and disease.

Condition	Doppler index
Normal	Over 1.0
Ischaemia	Under 1.0
Claudication	0.5 to 0.6
Rest pain	0.25
Gangrene	0.05

Aortography can be performed by the translumbar or retrograde femoral routes, the former requiring general anaesthesia. The choice depends largely on the patency of the iliac arteries. Special views of the origin of the profunda femoris are useful as it is commonly stenosed, although it may appear normal with standard views. In some cases a simple femoral arteriogram is all that is required.

The arteriogram will show the approximate extent of the disease process in terms of irregularity of the lumen, stenoses, occlusions, and the state of the distal arterial tree or 'run-off'. An adequate 'run-off' is essential if a bypass graft is to remain patent; generally, two of the three lower leg arteries should be patent.

The main sites of atheroma are (Figures 12.8, 12.9):

Aortoiliac segment in over 30 per cent of cases
Superficial femoral artery in about 60 per cent
Multiple level disease in about 7 per cent
Profunda origin in about two-thirds of above.

The site of the main arterial occlusion or stenosis and the state of the 'run-off' determine the feasibility of arterial reconstruction. It should always be assumed that the underlying atheroma will prove to be more extensive than arteriography suggests. Selection of the best procedure for multi-level disease is often difficult, and depends on the site of the apparent or measured maximum resistance.

Specialized investigations (not in wide clinical use) include:

The ischaemic leg   129

Bidirectional Doppler ultrasound. This demonstrates forward and reversed flow and turbulence due to disease. Various methods of analysis exist.

Pulse volume recording. Waveforms are produced from pressure changes in a leg cuff with each pulse. Various methods of analysis exist.

Ultrasound imaging techniques. These produce flow maps in three planes comparable with arteriography. At present the techniques are used mainly for investigation of carotid disease.

Figure 12.8 Atheromatous obstruction of aortoiliac segment.

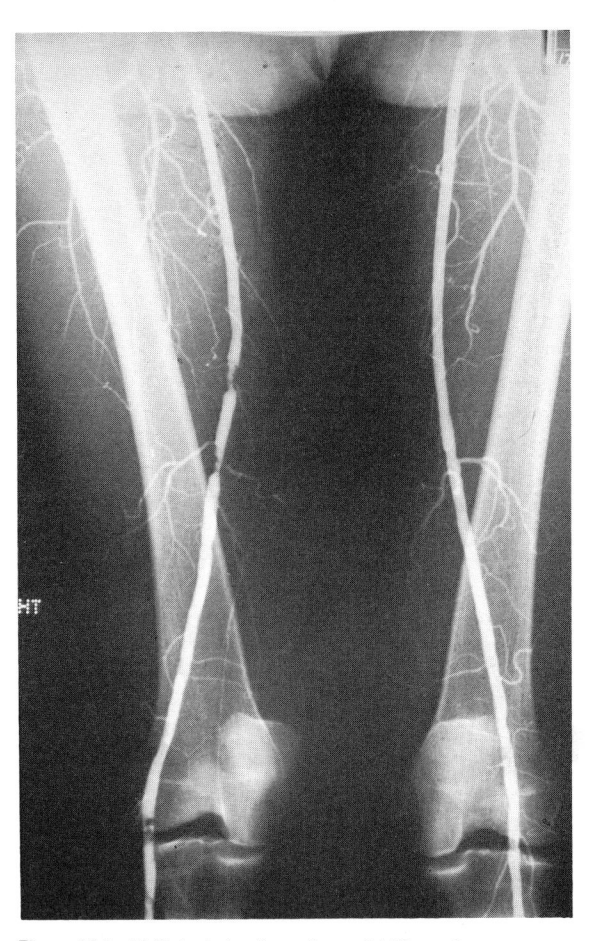

Figure 12.9 Multiple obstructions of superficial femoral artery.

Management of the ischaemic leg

Which cases should be referred to hospital? This depends on many factors but the general indications are given in Table 12.3.

The disability represented by claudication depends on many factors such as claudication distance, age and occupation of patient, and leisure interests. A man with exercise tolerance of 200 to 300 yards should not find his symptoms incapacitating unless his job entails much walking. Patients are often very unreliable in assessing their walking distance, and often a claimed distance of 25 to 50 yards is found to be 200 yards or more on careful questioning and observed performance.

Claudication may be more of a handicap in leisure activities such as golf or dancing than in the patient's job. Other conditions limiting exercise tolerance such as angina and dyspnoea are taken into account; there is little point in operating to relieve claudication if other factors are just as limiting.

Table 12.3 Indications for hospital referral.

Severe or progressive claudication, e.g. work suffering
Rest pain, necrosis or gangrene
Young patients with symptoms of aortoiliac disease
Patients with diabetic sepsis
Acutely ischaemic legs
Young patients, i.e. < 40 years, to rule out alternative disease.

Treatment

This is related to the natural history of the disease, i.e. atheroma. In general, patients presenting with claudication, as opposed to rest pain, have a fairly good prognosis. Roughly speaking, 50 per cent improve spontaneously, 40 per cent remain stable and only 10 per cent require surgical intervention. The treatment in this group is **conservative** unless exercise tolerance is so limited as to be incapacitating in terms of occupation or, less often, retirement activity.

Conservative treatment consists of:

- Regular exercise, i.e. walking, to encourage development of collaterals and improve claudication distance.
- Reassurance that the pain is not harmful and one can 'walk into it' with potential benefit.
- Avoidance of smoking; simple factual explanation of nature of disease and prognosis will often convince a patient.
- Weight reduction; this is advisable in obesity to reduce muscle work. (In practice it may be difficult while attempting also to stop smoking.)
- Raising the heels of the shoes; a heel raise of ½ to ¾ inch will reduce the work of calf muscles, and may improve walking distance.

> Vasodilator drugs have no place in the treatment of claudication alone. Reassurance and advice are cheaper, simpler and equally, if not more, effective.

Vasodilator drugs have no place in the treatment of claudication. They are incapable of improving blood flow through diseased vessels but they may **reduce** flow in the affected limb by diverting blood supply elsewhere. Despite this they are still widely supplied in claudicants, perhaps largely because of a desire to offer some form of treatment. Simple advice is both cheaper and equally effective.

Roughly half the patients presenting with claudication show a spontaneous improvement in exercise tolerance and only about one in ten deteriorate sufficiently to require surgery ultimately.

The prognosis is better for femoropopliteal disease than aortoiliac disease.

Operative treatment

Patients presenting with rest pain and/or necrosis require careful assessment with a view to arterial reconstruction. Similarly severe claudicants, young ischaemics and those with embolic episodes from aortic disease generally need surgery. Patients with claudication alone who cannot or will not stop smoking are not offered surgery.

Extensive gangrene of the foot invites amputation at some level. Other reasons for advising immediate amputation rather than reconstruction include severe cardio-pulmonary disease (threat to life and restricting activity), severe cerebrovascular disease, and paralysis of the relevant limb. Localized painless dry senile gangrene of one or two toes may be managed conservatively in the elderly patient. Occasionally satisfactory healing follows shedding of necrotic areas and even spontaneous amputation of a toe.

The management of the ischaemic leg is outlined in the flow chart (Figure 12.10). **It is a good guiding rule that only those patients who need and are fit to undergo arterial reconstruction require full investigation with aortography.** The procedure is invasive and carries a significant morbidity.

Operations available to revascularize lower limb

Proximal reconstruction

1. *Aortobifemoral bypass graft* using Dacron bifurcation (or 'trouser') graft from infrarenal aorta to common femoral arteries. It is occasionally combined with a distal type of bypass.
2. *Aortoiliac endarterectomy.* This is suitable for *localized* atheroma of aortic bifurcation and common iliac arteries.
3. *Iliofemoral or iliopopliteal bypass,* via extraperitoneal approach. Useful for unilateral

ischaemia avoiding a full aortic procedure.
4. *Profundaplasty.* This is a widening of the profunda origin as a single procedure (by patch grafting or endarterectomy), or as part of an aortobifemoral graft procedure. Suitable when the origin is stenosed but the distal profunda reasonably healthy.

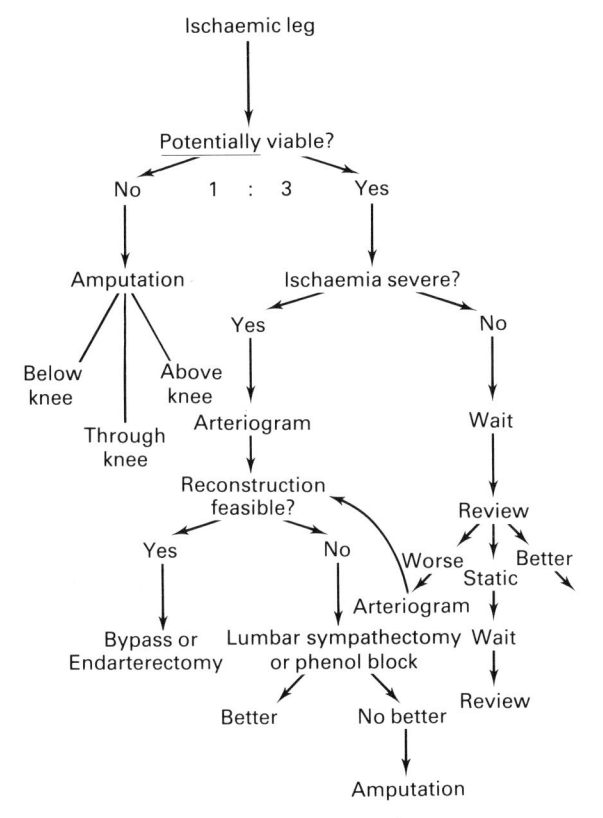

Figure 12.10 Management of the ischaemic leg.

Distal reconstruction
1. *Femoropopliteal bypass graft,* using autogenous long saphenous vein (reversed because of valves) from common femoral to distal popliteal artery. Alternative prosthetic materials such as Dacron, human umbilical vein and polytetrafluoroethylene may be used when autogenous vein is not available.
2. *Femoral endarterectomy* for proximal part of a superficial femoral artery, combined with technically superior vein bypass graft. Useful when only *limited* length of vein is available.
3. *Femorodistal bypass.* A long bypass to the tibial or peroneal artery in the distal calf, using in-situ long saphenous vein (with valves destroyed) or prosthetic graft. Results are inferior to those of femoropopliteal bypass.

Other procedures
1. *Lumbar sympathectomy* by transabdominal extraperitoneal route. Improves blood supply indirectly by eliminating vasomotor tone. Usually performed as supplement to bypass grafting to enhance flow through graft and make the best of distal perfusion. Alone it may be effective in relieving rest pain without necrosis or gangrene, where reconstruction is not practicable.
2. *Extra-anatomic (or cross over) bypass grafts* – axillofemoral and femorofemoral. Useful in revascularizing legs when abdominal surgery is impracticable. Subcutaneous route is used.

Any significant stenosis of the aortoiliac segment must be attended to before performing any distal bypass procedure, or the latter may undergo thrombosis due to slow flow, i.e. poor 'run-in'.

Most of these arterial reconstructions will be supplemented by lumbar sympathectomy, and excision of areas of irreversible necrosis (often digital amputation), to promote healing while the blood supply is maximal. Later graft failure may not then be followed by breakdown at such sites. The results of such procedures are summarized in Table 12.4.

Table 12.4 Comparison between different reconstructive procedures. (From Taylor, 1973).

	Mortality (%)	*Morbidity/ early graft failure* (%)	*5-year patency* (%)
Aortoiliac surgery	5	30	75
Femoro-popliteal bypass	1	7	50

The relatively poor patency rate for femoropopliteal grafts suggests that such procedures should be used more for limb salvage than for relief of claudication. All patients should be followed up after reconstruction.

Patients whose arteriogram findings rule out reconstruction are considered for **lumbar sympathectomy.** In elderly, poor-risk patients this may be effected by non-operative means with a phenol sympathetic block. Sympathectomy will not be sufficient in patients with necrosis or gangrene, and major amputation may be required. Before this decision is made, all other options should be considered. These include less severe procedures such as profundaplasty, femoro-femoral grafts and **percutaneous transluminal angioplasty (PTA)**. This is performed under local anaesthetic; it consists of passing dilating catheters into and through stenotic segments and inflating the catheters to break down the tough atherosclerotic plaque material. It is most effective for short stenoses in major vessels such as the iliacs and superficial femoral, but it has been used at all main sites of arterial disease. It is not as successful as reconstruction in the long term but is readily repeated. It may be used to improve flow through the iliac segment before a distal bypass.

Patients with critical ischaemia not suitable for bypass surgery and not relieved by sympathectomy face a major amputation. Certain **conservative measures** may yet be helpful in avoiding amputation, and indeed these form the mainstay of treatment for rest pain during investigation:

Analgesics, with potency according to the severity of the pain.
Elevation of the head end of the bed on blocks to improve perfusion of a foot.
Provision of a bed cradle.
Avoidance of direct or excessive heat.
Protection of painful areas of the foot with a light slipper or plastozote sandal.
Lambswool insulation of the toes.
Care of ischaemic lesions – cleaning; light dressings; Savlon powder; E.45 cream to calluses.
Drug treatment – certain agents such as beta blockers are often harmful and may need to be changed. There is no convincing benefit from vasoactive drugs, although many are on trial. Alcohol is useful for rest pain – it has vasodilator, analgesic, and sedative effects. Quinine sulphate is helpful for night cramps.

Amputation levels

Major amputation is usually performed at, above, or below knee level, but conservative procedures are adopted where possible:

Digital amputation – one or more toes, usually through metatarsophalangeal joint.
Transmetatarsal – loss of all toes with forefoot stump.
Symes amputation – at ankle level; this is useful in diabetes where the blood supply is satisfactory down to this level. Not popular in United Kingdom.
Below-knee; a functional knee joint is a great advantage in mobility. A long posterior flap technique is used.
Knee level – through the knee, Gritti-Stokes, supracondylar, etc. These provide a long lever, but it is awkward to fit an artificial limb and the technique has little advantage except for a double-amputee.
Above-knee – still the most common major amputation. Healing is most sure.

Rehabilitation after amputation

Most patients should be given an opportunity to try an artificial limb, but some are better suited to the use of a wheelchair from the outset. Physiotherapy is vital for preserving joint function and to increase mobility on one leg. A pneumatic pylon is useful in regaining balance and mobility at an early stage.

Unfortunately, a large proportion of amputees (about 5 per cent) come to a second amputation within months, and about half the lower-limb amputees die within two years. Follow-up should be continued as for other vascular cases, keeping a careful watch on the surviving limb. Phantom pain or paraesthesiae may be troublesome and require assessment by a pain specialist.

Acute ischaemia

The acutely ischaemic leg is a surgical emergency requiring immediate admission to hospital for assessment. The main causes are emboli, thrombosis and trauma. The onset is usually sudden and may occur during inpatient care for a different condition, particularly coronary thrombosis.

Arterial embolism

Both legs may be affected, due to 'saddle embolus' of the aortic bifurcation or bilateral leg embolization. The most common sites affected are shown in Figure 12.11. The pain and pallor normally leads to a rapid diagnosis, but associated numbness and loss of motor function can mimic hemiparesis, resulting in delayed referral. Other acute symptoms may suggest embolism to brain, arm or abdominal viscera.

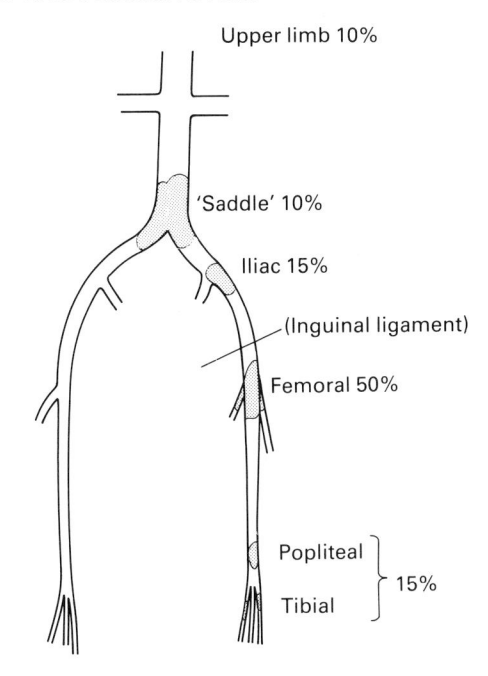

Figure 12.11 The main sites of arterial embolism.

- Upper limb 10%
- 'Saddle' 10%
- Iliac 15%
- (Inguinal ligament)
- Femoral 50%
- Popliteal / Tibial 15%

The source of embolism is the heart in about 90 per cent of cases but aortic atheroma and/or aneurysm may be responsible. If the onset is insidious and relatively painless, one should suspect **acute on chronic ischaemia** due to thrombosis, rather than embolism, of an already diseased arterial system. There is not always a history of claudication preceding the event as exercise tolerance may have been limited by other factors.

Any information on the patient's previous peripheral pulse status may be very helpful in distinguishing between an embolus and acute thrombosis of a stenosed segment in a major artery. For this reason full assessment of all peripheral pulses should be part of the normal examination for patients admitted with coronary thrombosis or atrial fibrillation. If the evidence favours embolism, emergency exploration of the artery is indicated; otherwise it is wise to obtain arteriograms first.

Arterial embolectomy

This is an emergency procedure, and should be carried out, if possible within 4 to 6 hours of onset. Local anaesthesia preferable for elderly, frail patients with past or recent history of coronary disease. Performed via the femoral artery in the groin for any level of 'blockage'.

Bilateral femoral approach for saddle embolus:
Procedure:

- All embolus and consequent thrombus is extracted with a Fogarty balloon catheter passed to ankle level.
- Profunda is also explored.
- Full anticoagulation with heparin is usually started either before or during the operation.
- Anticoagulation is continued with warfarin to treat the underlying cause (occasionally a further embolus occurs shortly after successful treatment, from a pre-existing source).
- Liberal fasciotomy of the lower leg should be performed in late explorations.

If the exploration reveals a thrombosed atheromatous femoral artery, effective clearance **may** be achieved with an embolectomy catheter, but arterial reconstruction is generally required and this is seldom performed as an emergency procedure without arteriography. In this situation the degree of ischaemia may be moderate rather than severe, and stable rather than deteriorating, so conservative treatment using low-molecular-weight dextran (Rheomacrodex) is more appropriate from the outset.

Early operation, within twelve hours and preferably within six hours, usually gives a good prognosis for life and limb, and it is worth performing embolectomy at any stage provided that the limb remains viable and the patient's general condition warrants it.

If symptoms are not severe and the popliteal pulse is present there may be little to gain from surgery. In this situation function is all important, and if the calf muscles are both active and non-tender with minimal impairment of skin sensation, exploration can be avoided; otherwise embolectomy is best attempted. At the other extreme, a neglected case with extensive fixed discoloration or necrosis and established contracture of the calf muscles clearly requires amputation.

Acute ischaemia of a limb is a surgical emergency. Urgent referral for assessment is mandatory.

Traumatic acute ischaemia

Arterial injury may be open or closed

Open injuries
 Division or laceration
 Traumatic false aneurysm or pulsating haematoma
 Traumatic arteriovenous fistula

Closed injuries
 External distortion or compression
 Intimal tears
 Thrombosis
 Arterial spasm.

Most of these injuries will produce ischaemia distal to the site of damage, but closed injuries are the commonest cause of acute ischaemia following trauma to the leg. If the classical symptoms and signs of acute ischaemia develop following fracture or dislocation in the leg, and fail to improve within an hour or two of reduction, immediate exploration of the site is needed or the limb may be lost.

Arterial spasm must never be assumed to be the cause of ischaemia unless the artery has been exposed at operation and opened to exclude an intimal tear. More limbs are lost through failure to explore the vessels than any other cause. As in other causes of acute ischaemia, irreversible changes may occur within six hours.

Compound fractures will often require full exploration to allow reduction of the fracture and internal fixation. Arterial repair should probably be performed first despite the lack of stability. **Muscle compression syndrome** due to increased tension in the fascial compartments of the leg may result from haematoma or post-ischaemic muscle swelling. Early decompression is essential to relieve pressure on the main blood vessels, and on the muscles themselves.

The following surgical procedures are available:
 Removal of the source of external distortion or compression
 Patch arterioplasty – generally using vein.
 End-to-end anastomosis – this is suitable for short segments of damage.
 Autogenous vein graft – this is required for longer segments of damage.
 Fasciotomy
  subcutaneous
  full-thickness
  single or multiple
  fibulectomy for the deep compartment.

It is clearly essential that any arterial repair should be supported by immobilization of the fracture site generally, with internal fixation. Repair of the main vein may also be required.

The diabetic foot

Diabetes mellitus is commonly complicated by foot problems and patients may develop:

 Neuropathic ulcers
 Sepsis
 Moist gangrene.

The ball of the foot under the first metatarsal head is a common site, but the heel or a bunion may be affected. The earliest lesion deep to the skin may remain in check for months or years. However, sepsis can develop very rapidly and spread through the tissues of the foot in a most destructive way.
 Treatment consists of:

 Control of diabetes generally with insulin
 Broad-spectrum antibiotics
 Surgical drainage and debridement.

Surgery has to be very thorough and radical to control diabetic sepsis and it may entail amputation of toes, 'ray' amputation deep into the foot, transmetatarsal amputation, and in all cases wide clearance of the affected skin and subcutaneous tissue, with healing by granulation. Simple drainage is usually doomed to failure.

If there is underlying ischaemia with loss of pulses in addition to the intrinsic diabetic problem, management follows the pattern outlined above for the chronically ischaemic leg. Unfortunately the distal, diabetic type of small-artery disease leaves little effective 'run-off' to support a bypass, so amputation is a common outcome. Sympathectomy is seldom helpful, because pre-existing neuropathy produces autosympathectomy.

> Diabetic foot sepsis must be treated quickly and radically to gain control.

Buerger's disease. This does not usually lend itself to reconstruction because of diffuse distal small vessel disease, i.e. poor 'run-off', but lumbar sympathectomy may help. Amputation is commonly required.

Senile gangrene. This is a form of dry, mummifying gangrene of the foot in elderly patients. Often the tips of several toes are involved. This condition may be remarkably painless, in which case little active treatment is required. If infection or severe pain supervene, either arterial reconstruction or amputation will be required. Generally, demarcation of gangrene is seen and patches of necrosis and even whole toes may separate spontaneously.

Patients with severe ischaemia usually have atheroma at other sites, and are elderly with limited life expectancy. The decision as to the most appropriate form of treatment is often difficult, taking into account the general health of the patient, his job and life-style, and the outlook for any bypass graft. Despite the length of some of the vascular operations, patients often tolerate them remarkably well and in most cases would naturally prefer to avoid amputation. Similarly, a pre-existing amputation on one side should not necessarily adversely affect the decision as to the place for reconstruction for the remaining leg. Life as a double amputee is much more difficult, whether or not artificial limbs are used.

Follow up

Hospital follow up is usual for untreated claudicants, patients undergoing reconstruction, and amputees. Further occlusive problems may arise in untreated legs and in grafts, for which additional surgery may be appropriate.

Acknowledgement

We wish to thank the Department of Medical Illustration, St Bartholomew's Hospital, London, for Figures 4, 5, 6, 8 and 9.

Reference

Taylor, G. W. (1973). Chronic arterial occlusion. In: *Peripheral Vascular Surgery* Ed. M. Birnstingl, pp. 219–221. London: Heinemann.

Index

Index

Abdominal
   acute pain 5–6, 68–73
   recurrent pain 6
Abscesses 7
Acquired hernia 80
Acute
   abdomen 5, 68–73
   cholecystitis 76
   ischaemia 126, 132–4
   lymph node pain 39–40
   mastoiditis 17
   otitis 15
   scrotal swelling 86–8
Adenoidectomy 33
Alternative medicine 110
Ampulla of Vater carcinoma 100
Amputation, leg 132
Appendicitis 5
Arterial embolism 132–3 ascites 97
Atherosclerosis 123
Autoimmune thyroiditis 51

Balanitis 11
Benign paroxysmal positional vertigo 23
Beta-adrenergic blockade 54
Bile-duct
   carcinoma 100
   secondary deposits 100
   stone 99
   stricture 95, 100
Biliary colic 73
Blood count 97
Bowel obstruction 6
Branchial
   cyst 43
   fistula 12
Breast
   abscess 67
   carcinoma 59–64
   examination 58
   screening 64
   unilateral development 66

Buerger's disease 135
Burns 7–8
Bypass grafts 130–31

Calculus, submandibular 45
Caldwell–Luc operation 33
Carbimazole 54–5
Carotid
   aneurysm 44
   body tumour 43
   tortuous artery 44
CAT *see* computer-assisted tomography
Catarrh 34
Cervical
   lymphadenopathy 39
   rib 45
Chillblains 126
Choledochus cyst 95
Cholesteatoma 19, 26
Chronic
   abdomen 6, 73–7
   epididymo-orchitis 90
   laryngitis 34
   lymph nodes 40
   mastitis 58
   nasal obstruction 29
   pancreatitis 76
   pharyngitis 34
   sinusitis 31
   suppurative otitis media 18
Chymopapain 109
Circumcision 11
Claudication distance 125
Cleft palate 13–14
Collaboration with surgeon 1–3
Collateral circulation 125
Colon carcinoma 77
Computer-assisted tomography 98
Conductive deafness 20–21
Congenital
   biliary atresia 95
   hernia 80

hypertrophic pyloric stenosis 7
Costochondritis 67
Cough 35
  test 117
Courvoisier's
  law 97
  sign 76
Crohn's disease 76
Cystic hygroma 13, 44
Cytotoxic therapy 63–4

Dermoid
  cysts 43
    external angular 12
Deviated nasal septum 31
Diabetic foot 134–5
Discogenic pain 109
Distal reconstruction 131
Diverticular disease 77
Doppler index 128
Dyspepsia 74
Dysphagia 75

Earache 15–18
Eczema, varicose 115
Elective admissions 8–14
Emergency admissions 4–8
Endolymphatic sac decompression 25
Enuresis 9
Epididymal cysts 88
Epigastric hernia 9
Epispadias 11
Ethmoid nasal polyps 29, 31
Euthyroid patient 52
External compression of varicosities 119

Facial palsy 19, 25–8
Fat necrosis 66
Femoral hernia 66
Fibroadenoma 65–6
Fibroadenosis 58–9
Fluctuating hearing loss 24
Foot, diabetic 134–5
Fournier's gangrene 91
Free thyroxine index 50
FTI *see* free thyroxine index

Gallstones 76, 93, 94–5
Gangrene 130
Genito-urinary conditions 9–12
Glue ears 16–17

Goitre 38, 51–2
Graves' disease 53–6
Grommets 16–17
Gynaecological acute abdomen 69

Haemangioma 13
Haematocele 87–8
Hare lip 13–14
Hashimoto's disease 51
Head injuries 4–5
Hepatitis B 96
Hepatocellular jaundice 94
Hernia 8–9
Hiatus hernia 75
Hodgkin's lymphomas 41
Hydrocele 9, 88
Hygroma, cystic 13, 44
Hyperthyroidism 47
Hypospadias 10
Hypothyroidism 48

IBS *see* irritable bowel syndrome
Incarcerated hernia 8
Inguinal hernia 8, 9, 94
Injection sclerotherapy 119
Intermittent claudication 125
Intranasal antrostomy 33
Intussusception 6
Inverted nipple 67
Iodine 48–9
  radioactive 55–6
Irritable bowel syndrome 77

Jerk nystagmus 24

Lactation cysts 65
Larynx
  chronic inflammation 34
  malignant disease 36
Leg
  arterial system 124
  venous system 112
Leriche's syndrome 125
Ligations 120
Littre's hernia 78
Liver
  failure 96
  tumours 94
Lumbar sympathectomy 131–2
Lymph nodes 38
  acute painful 39–40

chronic 40
  metastatic 40
Lymphadenopathy 13
  cervical 39
Lymphatic cysts 44
Lymphoproliferative disease 41

Mammary duct ectasia 67
Mammography 60, 64
Mastoidectomy 20
Mastoiditis 17
Mechanical back pain 102, 109
Meckel's diverticulum 6
Medicolegal back pain 105
Menière's disease 24
Mesenteric arteries 76
Metastatic
  glands in portal hepatitis 95
  lymph nodes 40

Naevi 13
Neonate
  plasma volume 4
  vomiting 6–7
Newborn *see* neonate
Nipple
  discharge 66
  inverted 67

Obstruction
  abdominal 72
  intrahepatic 94
  nasal 29–31
  urinary tract 10
Obturator hernia 79, 84
Oesophagitis 75
OGD *see* oral gastroduodenoscopy
Oöphorectomy 63
Oral gastroduodenoscopy 98
Orchidectomy 91
Orchidopexy 12
Otitis 15–16, 18

Pain clinics 110
Pancoast's tumour 45
Pancreas
  arteriogram 88
  carcinoma 76, 95, 100
Paranasal sinus malignancies 35

Paraphimosis 11
Parasitic infection 95
Parotid swelling 12
Paterson-Kelly syndrome 37
Penis, abnormalities 10–11
Peptic ulcer 75
Percutaneous
  transhepatic cholangiography 98
  transluminal angioplasty 132
Perforation of eardrum 18
Peri-areolar inflammation 66
Perimenopausal cysts 64–5
Peritonism 73
Perthe's test 118
Pharynx
  chronic inflammation 34
  malignant tumours 37
Phimosis 11
Physiological goitre 51
Plasma volume, neonates 4
Positional testing 23
Postcricoid carcinoma 37
Postnasal
  carcinoma 35–6
  drip 34
Pre-hepatic jaundice 94
Primary varicose veins 112
Proctitis 77
Propranolol 54
Prosthesis, breast 62
Prothrombin time 97
Proximal reconstruction 130
PTA *see* percutaneous transluminal angioplasty
PTC *see* percutaneous transhepatic cholangiography
Pyloric stenosis, congenital hypertrophic 7
Pyriform fossa tumours 37

Radioactive iodine 55
Ranula 12
Rectum, carcinoma 77
Recurrent abdominal pain 6
Reflux oesophagitis 75
Refractory venous ulcers 121
Rhinitis medicamentosa 30
Rhizotomy 109
Richter's hernia 78

Salivary gland disorders 45
Schirmer's test 26
Sclerosing cholangitis 95, 100
Sclerotherapy 119
Secondary varicose veins 113

Sensorineuronal deafness 21–2
Serum
  alkaline phosphatase 97
  bilirubin 97
  T_3 50
  T_4 49–50
  TSH 49
Sialogram 45
Sickle-cell disease 95
Sigmoidoscopy 77
Singer's nodes 34
Sliding hernia 84
Spermatocele 59
Spine
  adolescent 103
  pathology 104, 109
Spondylolisthesis 103
Steroid-receptor measurement 64
Stomach, carcinoma 75
Sturge–Kalischer-Weber syndrome 13
Submandibular swellings 45–6
Submucous resection of nasal septum 31
Subperiostal abscess 17

TBG *see* thyroid binding globulin
Testis
  torsion 54
  tumours 90
  undescended 11–12
Thrombophlebitis, superficial 115
Thyroglossal cyst 12, 42
Thyroid
  binding globulin 49
  cysts 52
  function investigation 48–50
  malignancy 51, 52–3
  nodule 50–51
  swellings 42
Thyrotoxicosis 52, 53–6
Thyrotrophin
  -releasing hormone 49
  -stimulating hormone 49
Tonsillectomy 33
Torsion, testicular 87
Tourniquet tests 117–18
Transaminase 97
Traumatic acute ischaemia 134
Trendelenburg procedure 120
TRH *see* thyrotrophin-releasing hormone
TSH *see* thyrotrophin-stimulating hormone

Ulcers
  refractory venous 121
  varicose 116
Ultrasound scan 98
Umbilical hernia 9
Ureteric colic 72
Urinary tract infections 10
Urine, bilirubin 97
UTI *see* urinary tract infections

Varicocele 88
Vasomotor rhinitis 29
Vertigo 19, 22–5
Vesicoureteric reflex 10
Vestibular failure 23
Vomiting, neonatal 6–7

Wharton's duct obstruction 45
Whipple's operation 100